Twelve-Lead Electrocardiography for ACLS Providers

D. BRUCE FOSTER, D.O.

Chief, Department of Emergency Medicine
Waynesboro Hospital
Waynesboro, Pennsylvania

W.B. SAUNDERS COMPANY
A Division of Harcourt Brace & Company
PHILADELPHIA LONDON TORONTO
MONTREAL SYDNEY TOKYO

W.B. SAUNDERS COMPANY
A Division of Harcourt Brace & Company
The Curtis Center
Independence Square West
Philadelphia, Pennsylvania 19106

Library of Congress Cataloging-in-Publication Data

Foster, D. Bruce.
   Twelve-lead electrocardiography for ACLS providers / D. Bruce
Foster. — 1st ed.
     p.   cm.
   ISBN 0–7216–5873–3
   1. Electrocardiography. I. Title.
   DNLM: 1. Electrocardiography—methods. 2. Heart Diseases—
diagnosis. WG 140 F754t 1996
RC683.5.E5F63 1996
616.1′207547—dc20
DNLM/DLC   95–25164

TWELVE-LEAD ELECTROCARDIOGRAPHY FOR ACLS PROVIDERS   ISBN 0–7216–5873–3

Printed in the United States of America.

Last digit is the print number: 9   8   7   6   5   4   3   2   1

To my parents, Anne and Donald Foster,
who encouraged me to leave the world
a better place than I found it;

To Thaddeus Prout, M.D.,
retired Chief of Medicine
at the Greater Baltimore Medical Center
and Associate Professor of Medicine
at the Johns Hopkins University,
who provided me with a role model of
physician, scholar, and gentleman;

And to Jan, Brian, and Ali,
who have made life worth living.

Preface

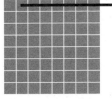

*T*welve-Lead Electrocardiography for ACLS Providers was written in response to a need for a clear, concise, introductory level text in the morphologic interpretation of electrocardiograms. It was developed primarily for nurses, paramedics, and physicians who are ACLS certified and are already familiar with cardiac dysrhythmias. The text therefore deals solely with morphology and does not discuss dysrhythmias.

The need for this text was spurred by the revolutionary development in the 1980s of thrombolytic therapy for acute myocardial infarction (AMI) and by the evolving importance of the role of critical care nurses, prehospital ALS providers, and emergency department physicians in the early recognition and treatment of AMI.

The text contains several very clinical chapters on the role of the ECG in the evaluation of chest pain and the selection of patients for thrombolytic therapy. I have tried to include all the pertinent information that ACLS providers working in emergency medical systems will need to know in order to implement chest pain evaluation protocols—and, I hope, to speed thrombolysis. In reality, however, the text should prove to be equally valuable to medical students and non–critical care physicians who need a working knowledge of the important fundamentals of morphologic electrocardiography, but who need not become professional electrocardiographers. Thus, the text emphasizes simplicity, clinically useful concepts, and common clinical parlance. It is written in a conversational tone and is not intended to serve as a reference text for serious postgraduate students of electrocardiography.

Nevertheless, fundamental electrophysiologic principles are emphasized to the extent that students have the opportunity to deduce patterns created by both physiologic and pathologic processes, rather than relying on memorizing ECG patterns of disease. I have tried, in the process, to communicate the sense of joy that comes from deduction and understanding, as opposed to the drudgery of memorization.

Many people played an important role in the writing of this text, primary among whom are the many students who have instructed me in what works and what doesn't work over the 15 years that I have taught electrocardiography. Special thanks are in order to Mr. Fred Bolland, Mr. Larry Berry, and the capable staff in the Cardiopulmonary Department of the Waynesboro Hospital for their tireless efforts in providing me with high-quality original tracings. My thanks go also to Dr. Rose Dagen of the Division of Cardiology for her help in procuring some of the rarer tracings and for her meticulous review of the manuscript. It is a better book because of her suggestions. Lauren Datcher, R.N., patiently spotted virtually every typo in the manuscript. And finally, I am indebted to Robert A. Mack, retired Professor at the Massachusetts Institute of Technology, whose computer expertise and unfailing availability made the critical technical aspects of this work possible.

D. Bruce Foster, D.O.

Notice

Electrocardiography is an ever-changing field. Standard safety precautions must be followed, but as new research and clinical experience broaden our knowledge, changes in treatment and drug therapy become necessary or appropriate. The editors of this work have carefully checked the generic and trade drug names and verified drug dosages to ensure that the dosage information in this work is accurate and in accord with the standards accepted at the time of publication. Readers are advised, however, to check the product information currently provided by the manufacturer of each drug to be administered to be certain that changes have not been made in the recommended dose or in the contraindications for administration. This is of particular importance in regard to new or infrequently used drugs. It is the responsibility of the treating physician, relying on experience and knowledge of the patient, to determine dosages and the best treatment for the patient. The editors cannot be responsible for misuse or misapplication of the material in this work.

THE PUBLISHER

Contents

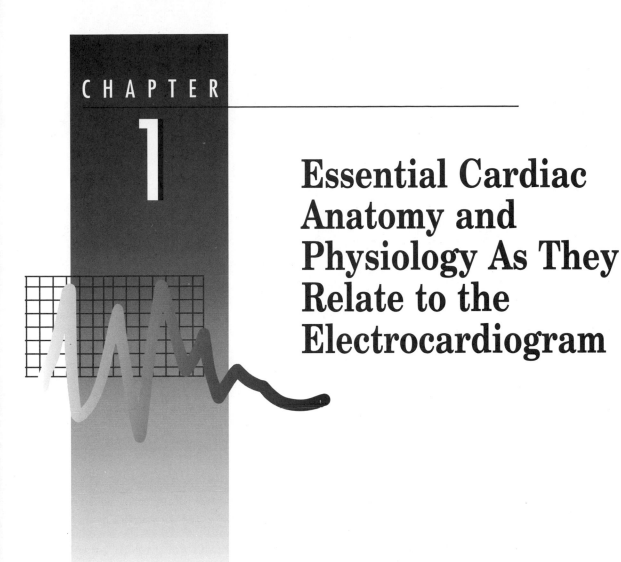

CHAPTER 1

Essential Cardiac Anatomy and Physiology As They Relate to the Electrocardiogram

Developing the capability of interpreting a 12-lead electrocardiogram (ECG) depends on an understanding of a few fundamental principles of anatomy and physiology. In this chapter, I will review the electrical conduction system of the heart and the methods used to record depolarization.

The Specialized Cardiac Conduction System

In the normal heart during sinus rhythm, impulse formation is initiated in the *sinoatrial (SA) node* (Fig. 1–1), and then spreads as a wave of depolarization over the atria until it reaches the *atrioventricular (AV) node,* near the junction of the interatrial and interventricular septa.

The AV node represents the sole pathway for conducting the impulse from the atria to the ventricles, except when it is bypassed by abnormal congenital pathways. Its unique purpose is to slow the rate of impulse conduction to give the atria time to finish emptying of blood and the ventricles time to finish filling with blood. This is necessary because mechanical contraction of cardiac muscle is normally slower than the rapid process of electrical depolarization (Fig. 1–2).

The *common bundle of His* next conducts the impulse through the superior ventricular septum and then quickly divides into the *right bundle branch* and *left bundle branch*. Perhaps because the left ventricle is bigger than the right ventricle, the left bundle branch splits into two *hemibundles,*

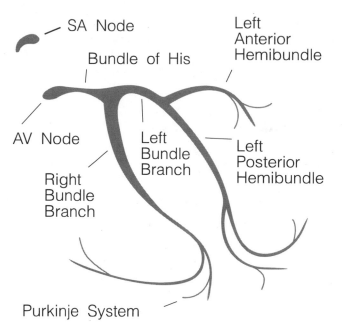

Figure 1–1
The specialized cardiac conduction system.

one running anteriorly and superiorly, as if out of the page toward the reader, and the other running posteriorly and inferiorly into the page, as if away from the reader.

Finally, the bundle branches divide numerous times into *Purkinje fibers* that are the final pathway for conduction of the impulse to ventricular muscle. Once ventricular muscle is stimulated by the impulse traveling down the Purkinje fibers, it depolarizes outwardly from *endocardium* to *epicardium*.

Electrical impulses are conducted much more rapidly through the specialized conduction system of the heart just described above than through typical cardiac muscle. This allows the electrical impulse to reach almost all of ventricular muscle nearly simultaneously, thus allowing for coordinated contraction of the ventricles. There is a small but important difference in the *sequence of activation* of various portions of the ventricles, which will be discussed later.

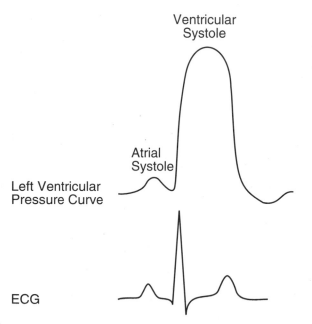

Figure 1–2
Synchronous recording of left ventricular pressure curve and ECG. The time required for mechanical contraction during atrial and ventricular systole is shown by the pressure curve. Note how these times exceed the times required for atrial and ventricular depolarization (P wave and QRS duration).

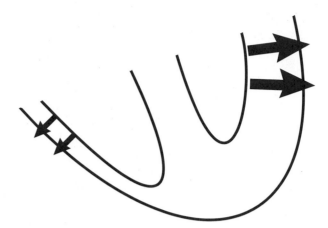

Figure 1–3
Schematic drawing showing greater thickness of the septum and wall of the left ventricle as compared with the right ventricle. Arrows represent force vectors, illustrating that as a result of its greater thickness, the left ventricle generates greater voltages.

Muscle Mass of Cardiac Chambers

The atria pump blood only very short distances (across the AV valves into the ventricles); therefore, they are very thin-walled structures with very little muscle mass. Conversely, the right ventricle must pump blood all the way through the lungs and therefore has a thicker wall and more muscle mass. Finally, the left ventricle pumps blood out to the entire body and therefore has the thickest wall of all the chambers, three to four times thicker than the wall of the right ventricle (Fig. 1–3).

One of the determinants of the size of an electrical complex on the ECG is how much voltage is generated by depolarization of a given portion of the heart. Thus, the QRS is normally larger than the P wave because depolarization of the greater muscle mass of the ventricles generates more voltage than does depolarization of the thinner walls of the atria.

Recording a Wave of Depolarization

A wave of depolarization spreading across a strip of muscle can be recorded by a *galvanometer,* an instrument that measures voltage. Figure 1–4 illustrates an isolated strip of muscle that is stimulated at the left end, producing a wave of depolarization that spreads from left to right. Three electrodes placed on this muscle strip are connected to a galvanometer. The needle of the galvanometer

Figure 1–4
Strip chart recording of depolarization of an isolated muscle strip "viewed" by three exploring electrodes. As the wave of depolarization comes toward each electrode, it produces a positive deflection on the recording. As the wave passes under the electrode, the needle begins to swing down toward neutral, then inscribes a clearly negative deflection as the wave begins to go away from the electrode.

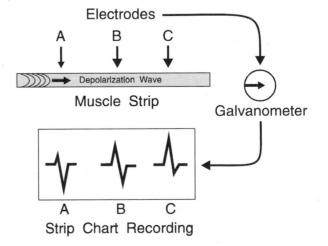

swings up or down as the electrical events in the muscle strip are measured. These events can then be permanently recorded by attaching a pen to the end of the needle and passing a paper strip at a constant speed beneath the pen. The result is called a *strip chart recording.*

By convention, the needle swings up when an impulse is coming toward a measuring electrode and down when an impulse is going away from an electrode. Note that as the wave of depolarization in Figure 1–4 comes toward each electrode, there is an initial positive deflection seen on the corresponding recording of the strip chart. As the wave passes directly beneath each electrode for an instant, the wave is going neither toward nor away from the electrode; therefore, the needle rapidly swings down toward the neutral position. However, the wave doesn't really stop but continues to move, immediately passing the electrode and then going away from it. This causes the needle to continue downward past the neutral position to record a negative deflection. When the wave finally reaches the end of the muscle strip and depolarization is over, the needle again swings up to the neutral position and comes to rest on what is called the *isoelectric line.*

Note in Figure 1–4 that strip chart recordings A, B, and C look slightly different, depending on the position from which their electrodes "viewed" the spreading wave of depolarization. Since most of the time the wave of depolarization was spreading toward electrode C, the corresponding C recording is predominantly upright, with only a brief negative deflection at the end. Conversely, since most of the time the impulse was spreading away from electrode A, strip chart recording A is predominantly negative with only a brief initial period of positive deflection corresponding to the short time the impulse was coming toward electrode A. This simple concept of measuring voltages in muscle from different locations or "viewpoints" is the essence of 12-lead electrocardiography.

Electrocardiographic Waveforms

W hat I called strip chart recordings A, B, and C in the first chapter, I will now refer to in electrocardiographic (ECG) jargon as waveforms or complexes. This chapter reviews the electrical events in the heart that correspond to each complex, reviews the normal parameters for these complexes and the intervals between them, and finally, reviews waveform terminology.

The ECG Grid

The familiar ECG grid consists of squares of 1 mm (Fig. 2–1). As you know from your previous exposure to dysrhythmias, time is measured on the horizontal axis of the grid. Each small box, which measures 1 mm horizontally, equals 0.04 second in time. The width of ECG complexes is commonly referred to as *duration*.

You may also remember that the vertical axis is a relative measure of voltage but is usually expressed in millimeters of positive or negative deflection rather than in volts. The height or depth of deflection is commonly referred to as *amplitude*.

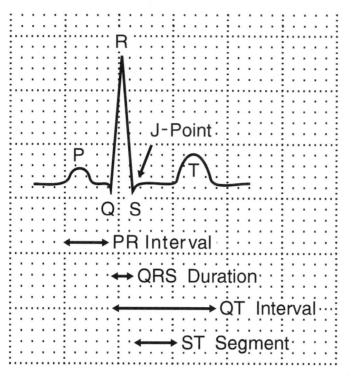

Figure 2–1
The ECG grid with waveforms and intervals. Each small box in the grid represents 0.04 second in time horizontally. The vertical axis measures relative voltage but is usually expressed in millimeters of amplitude.

The P Wave

The P wave, of course, corresponds to the depolarization of atrial muscle. Because there is relatively little atrial muscle mass, only low voltages are normally produced. The amplitude of the P wave should normally not exceed 2 or 3 mm, and its duration should not be greater than 0.11 second. Greater amplitude or duration may often indicate enlargement of the atria with more than the usual amount of muscle mass (Fig. 2–2).

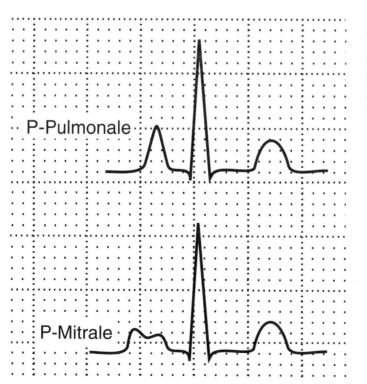

Figure 2–2
Two different kinds of P wave abnormalities seen in lead II. P-pulmonale with tall, peaked P waves is commonly seen in patients with right atrial enlargement secondary to pulmonary hypertension. P-mitrale, characterized by broad, notched P waves, is commonly seen in left atrial enlargement secondary to mitral valve disease.

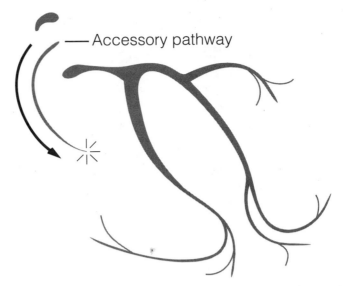

Accessory pathway

Figure 2–3
Schematic diagram of the specialized conduction system of
the heart showing a congenital accessory pathway from
atria to ventricles. The accessory pathway bypasses the
AV node and rapidly conducts the impulse directly to the
ventricles, producing early depolarization, or pre-
excitation.

The PR Interval

The PR interval corresponds to the time it takes an impulse to travel from
the SA node all the way down through the conduction system to the first muscle
fibers stimulated in the ventricles. Therefore, it is measured from the beginning
of the P wave to the beginning of the QRS. Note in Figure 2–1 that, although
you can see depolarization of the atria in the form of the P wave, you cannot
see the impulse traveling through the AV node, bundle of His, bundle branches,
or Purkinje fibers because the voltages in these structures are too low to register
on our galvanometer.

As you will remember from your study of dysrhythmias, the normal PR
interval runs from about 0.12 to 0.20 second. Shorter intervals indicate *accelerated conduction* from the atria to the ventricles, such as is seen in *Wolff-
Parkinson-White (WPW) syndrome* or in a junctional pacemaker, with which
you are already familiar from your study of dysrhythmias. In WPW syndrome
there are congenitally aberrant pathways (Fig. 2–3) outside the normal conduction system that bypass the slowing effect of the AV node and rapidly conduct
impulses from the atria directly to the ventricles—a kind of electrical "short
circuit" manifested by the classic *delta wave* (Fig. 2–4).

PR intervals longer than 0.20 second indicate a delay in normal conduction
somewhere in the conduction system between the AV node and the bifurcation
of the bundle of His—the familiar *first-degree AV block*.

Figure 2–4
Wolff-Parkinson-White (WPW) syndrome as seen in lead II.
Note that the ventricles are activated very early, as evidenced
by the delta wave beginning very shortly after the P wave.
Thus, the hallmark of WPW syndrome is a delta wave,
creating a very short PR interval.

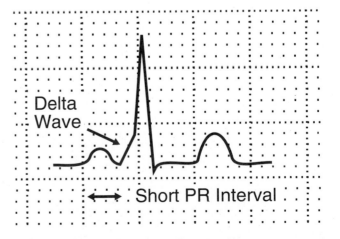

Delta
Wave

←→ Short PR Interval

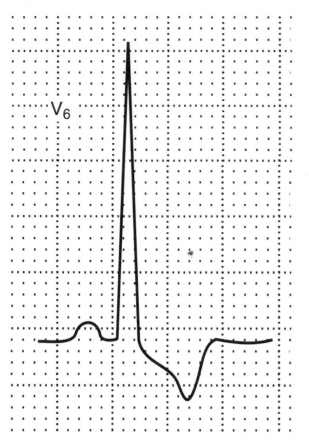

Figure 2–5
Left ventricular hypertrophy as seen in lead V₆. Note that the amplitude of the R wave exceeds 25 mm. The ST segment and the T wave show a typical "strain pattern" of LVH.

The QRS

The QRS is naturally the largest complex on the ECG because it corresponds to depolarization of the ventricles with their larger muscle mass. QRS amplitude may therefore normally reach as high as 25 mm or more (5 big boxes) in large individuals or in those with thin chest walls that actually allow the precordial electrodes to be closer to the heart. Amplitudes greater than 25 mm are frequently associated with *chamber enlargement* (ventricular hypertrophy) as seen in Figure 2–5. Conversely, very low QRS amplitudes are also abnormal and may be seen with diffuse, severe cardiac disease or with such illnesses as pericardial effusion and hypothyroidism.

If the conduction system is working properly, the duration of the QRS should be less than 0.10 second. Durations of 0.10 second or greater indicate a delay in the spread of depolarization through the ventricles—the so-called *intraventricular conduction delay,* such as is seen in bundle branch blocks (Fig. 2–6). More on that later.

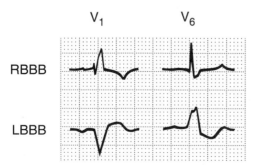

Figure 2–6
Two examples of bundle branch block. Note that the QRS duration is increased to 0.12 second or more and that there is deformity of the ST and T waves, with T waves usually inscribed in the opposite direction from the QRS. The characteristic RSR′ pattern is seen in V₁ and V₂ in right bundle branch block (RBBB) and in V₅ or V₆ in left bundle branch block (LBBB).

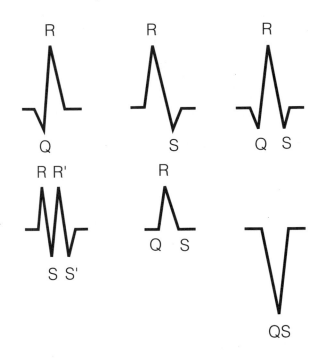

Figure 2–7
QRS nomenclature. Note that when the complex has no Q or S
wave, it is still permissible to call it a "QRS."

Later on, you will see that it becomes very important to be able to describe
the various combinations of positive and negative deflections of the QRS very
accurately. It is worthwhile therefore to spend a little time now reviewing
nomenclature of the QRS.

Figure 2–7 shows some of the various possible QRS inscription combinations. The rules are as follows:

1. The first deflection of the complex is called a *Q wave* if it is negative.
2. The first positive deflection of the complex is called an *R wave*.
3. A negative deflection coming after an R wave is called an *S wave*.
4. Positive deflections coming after the first R wave are labeled *R'* (*R prime*).
5. Negative deflections coming after the first S wave are labeled *S'* (*S prime*).

ST Segment

The ST segment represents the time between completion of depolarization
of the ventricles and the onset of repolarization of the ventricles. It is normally
isoelectric and gently blends into the upslope of the subsequent T wave (see
Fig. 2–1). The point at which the ST segment takes off from the QRS is called
the *J-point*.

The ST segment plays a very important role in the diagnosis of ischemic
heart disease, particularly in acute myocardial infarction (AMI). Most of you
are aware that dramatic *ST segment elevation* is one of the hallmarks of AMI
(Fig. 2–8). Sometimes, however, the ST segment may be slightly elevated above
the base line across the entire tracing in perfectly healthy people, particularly
young males. This finding is called *benign early repolarization changes* and
reflects a phase of repolarization of the ventricles that occurs earlier in the
cardiac cycle than in most people.

The ST segment can also be *depressed* below the base line in a variety of
conditions, such as ischemia and ventricular hypertrophy. ST segment shifts
of all sorts will be discussed in detail in later chapters.

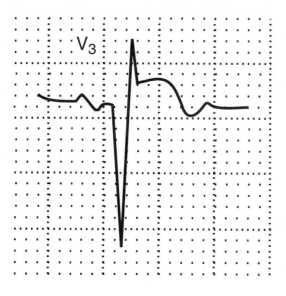

Figure 2–8
The three hallmarks of acute myocardial infarction, including ST segment elevation, T wave inversion, and Q wave formation.

The T Wave

The T wave corresponds to repolarization of the ventricles. It is normally inscribed in the same direction as the predominant deflection of the QRS and has less amplitude than the QRS. Abnormalities of the T wave predominantly take the form of *inversion* (being inscribed in the opposite direction to the QRS), as we have seen in bundle branch block, left ventricular hypertrophy, and AMI. They may also take the form of very large or very small amplitudes, as in hyperkalemia and hypokalemia (Fig. 2–9).

The QT Interval

The QT interval is measured from the beginning of the QRS to the end of the T wave, and normal intervals vary with heart rate and the person's sex. Therefore, when determining whether a QT interval is normal or not, it is best to use a chart that plots normal intervals against heart rate and sex (Table 2–1).

The primary potential abnormality of the QT interval is *prolongation,* reflecting delays in ventricular repolarization. This is commonly the result of administration of drugs, such as procainamide or quinidine, or electrolyte

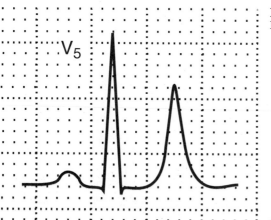

Figure 2–9
Extremely tall, pointed T waves seen with hyperkalemia.

■ **Table 2–1 Normal QT Intervals**

Heart Rate	Normal		Upper Limits Normal	
	Men & Children	Women	Men	Women
40	0.449	0.461	0.491	0.503
43	0.438	0.450	0.479	0.479
46	0.426	0.438	0.466	0.478
48	0.420	0.432	0.460	0.471
50	0.414	0.425	0.453	0.464
52	0.407	0.418	0.445	0.456
54.5	0.400	0.411	0.438	0.449
57	0.393	0.404	0.430	0.441
60	0.386	0.396	0.422	0.432
63	0.378	0.388	0.413	0.423
66.5	0.370	0.380	0.404	0.414
70.5	0.361	0.371	0.395	0.405
75	0.352	0.362	0.384	0.394
80	0.342	0.352	0.374	0.384
86	0.332	0.341	0.363	0.372
92.5	0.321	0.330	0.351	0.360
100	0.310	0.318	0.338	0.347
109	0.297	0.305	0.325	0.333
120	0.283	0.291	0.310	0.317
133	0.268	0.276	0.294	0.301
150	0.252	0.258	0.275	0.282
172	0.234	0.240	0.255	0.262

From Ashman R, Hull E: *Essentials of Electrocardiography.* New York: The Macmillan Company, 1945. By permission.

imbalance, particularly as in hypocalcemia. When the QT interval is prolonged, there is a greater opportunity for R on T phenomenon and a higher incidence of ventricular reentry dysrhythmias and sudden death.

A Word About Nonspecific ST and T Wave Changes

Frequent readers of ECG reports will be frustratingly familiar with the term *nonspecific ST and T wave changes.* This term reflects the unfortunate reality that the ECG has significant limitations as a diagnostic tool and that there are many ECG abnormalities that have more than one cause and are therefore not specific for any one disease state. Thus, the term nonspecific has a genuine usefulness in calling the reader's attention to waveform changes that are abnormal but that cannot be ascribed to any single cause.

Cardiac Vectors and Lead Systems

In this chapter I will discuss the concept of vectors, the sequences of activation of heart muscle, and the directions from which various leads "look" at the heart. This will set the stage for figuring out what the normal ECG looks like in each lead and why.

Force Vectors

Undoubtedly you have heard it said in the past that wavefronts of depolarization really do not travel in straight lines but spread over tissue more like a ripple in a pond spreads out from the point into which you toss a stone. This is actually quite a good analogy but is difficult to illustrate in a diagram. It has always been easier to describe the direction in which a wave is traveling and the magnitude of its force (in this case voltage) by using arrows.

Thus in Figure 3–1, we see an attempt to depict a wavefront of depolarization (spreading from endocardium to epicardium) with both curved lines, representing the spreading edge of the wavefront, and short arrows, representing both the direction in which the wavefront is traveling and its relative force (voltage). These arrows are called *force vectors*.

If we mentally eliminate the curved lines and keep just the arrows to represent the wavefront, we can easily see that the sum of all the little arrows can be represented by the one larger arrow in the middle of the diagram. This larger arrow represents the *mean* direction of the wavefront

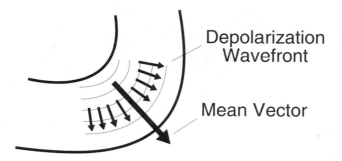

Figure 3–1
Schematic section through a ventricle showing the spread of a wave of depolarization from endocardium to epicardium. The wavefront and its relative force is shown by the series of small arrows. The mean direction of the wavefront and its mean force is represented by the larger arrow.

and its relative force. It is called a *summation vector* because it represents the sum of all the little vectors. The larger the arrow, the greater the force.

Sequences of Depolarization

It is possible to create a simple illustration of the major sequences of depolarization of the heart and the relative voltages encountered by drawing a series of summation vectors (Fig. 3–2). It is also useful to describe the direction in which these vectors are traveling by superimposing our drawing on a 360-degree compass rose. We will modify our standard compass rose a little bit, however, by assigning the zero-degree mark to the horizontal on the right and going clockwise with positive degrees to +180° and counterclockwise with negative degrees to −180°. This is done by *convention* (by general agreement) in electrocardiography.

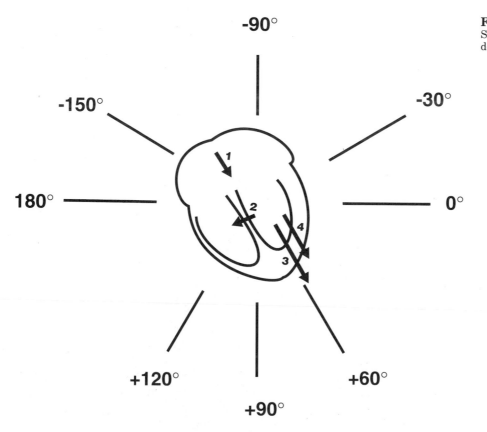

Figure 3–2
Summation vectors of cardiac depolarization.

Note in Figure 3–2 that vector 1 represents depolarization of the atria and that the wavefront spreads down over the atria toward the patient's left at roughly a 40- to 50-degree angle. This vector would obviously correspond to the P wave of the ECG.

Vector 2 represents depolarization of the ventricular septum, the first part of the ventricles to be activated, and corresponds to the first deflection of the QRS complex. Note that depolarization of the septum normally takes place from left to right. This is because the impulse normally travels somewhat faster down the left bundle branch than down the right bundle branch. Therefore, the left side of the septum is activated first.

Vector 3 represents the summation vector of depolarization of the bulk of ventricular muscle and therefore corresponds to the main deflection of the QRS. Note that this vector is normally angled slightly to the left at about 60°, despite the fact that depolarization of both ventricles is initiated almost simultaneously. This is so for three reasons. First, the considerably greater muscle mass of the left ventricular generates greater voltages than does the right ventricle, with the result that the summation vector is shifted leftward. Second, it takes more time for the wavefront to pass through the wall of the left ventricle than that of the right ventricle because of the considerably greater thickness of the left ventricular wall. This leaves the electrical forces in the left ventricle relatively unopposed during the later part of ventricular depolarization and thus also serves to shift the summation vector leftward. Finally, the position of the heart itself in the chest cavity is such that the apex is tilted slightly toward the left, as seen in Figure 3–3.

Vector 4 is the resultant of the electrical forces generated by repolarization of the ventricles and therefore is responsible for producing the T wave of the ECG. Because repolarization is a slower process than depolarization, the T wave does not have the same sharp configuration as the QRS. Vector 4 is generally inclined at about the same angle as the main vector of ventricular depolarization. Therefore, the inscription of the T wave on the ECG is usually in the same direction as the major deflection of the QRS.

Lead Systems

The exact placement of the leads in the standard 12-lead ECG is the result of general agreement that has evolved over the years among electrocardiographers. Many additional lead locations other than the usual are possible. We will avoid, however, a discussion of the actual physical placement of leads (e.g., Einthoven's triangle) because it is not necessary to your understanding of ECG morphology and frequently results in confusion. Suffice it to say that the simple description of lead systems given in the following paragraphs is entirely sufficient to support an accurate interpretation of the ECG.

We saw in Chapter 1 that the strip chart recordings of electrical events in a strip of muscle look different, depending upon the position of the electrode that views the events. The 12 leads of the standard 12-lead ECG were selected to offer a wide variety of "views" of the heart. Although oversimplified, the following description of the leads in the 12-lead ECG is a useful and clinically quite accurate method of conceptualizing lead systems.

The 12-lead ECG "looks" at the heart in two different planes (Fig. 3–3). The three so-called *standard limb leads* (I, II, and III) and the three so-called *augmented limb leads* (aVR, aVL, and aVF) all look at the heart from the "edges" of the *frontal plane* as if the body were flat or unidimensional. It is common practice to refer to all six leads, taken together, simply as the *limb leads.*

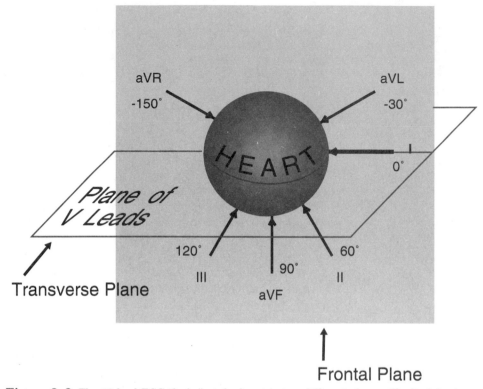

Figure 3–3. The 12-lead ECG "looks" at the heart in two different planes. The limb leads examine the heart in the frontal plane, and the V leads examine the heart in the transverse plane.

The six *V leads* (V_1 to V_6) across the precordium look at the heart in the horizontal or *transverse* plane (Fig. 3–5). These leads allow us to look at the front and left side of the heart and complete a more three-dimensional perspective.

Note in Figure 3–4 that in order to describe from which direction each of the limb leads looks at the heart in the frontal plane, we have again used our modified compass rose. It is useful to think of each lead as being an *exploring electrode* (an electrode that explores the heart) located in the positions shown in the figure. In actuality, of course, this is not the case. Rather, the electrocardiograph machine manipulates signals in its internal circuitry to give us tracings that look much as if electrodes were placed in those positions.

One can readily see then that lead aVR "looks down" on the heart from above and to the right at a position of $-150°$. Lead aVL looks down on the heart from above and to the left at $-30°$. Lead I looks at the heart on the horizontal directly from the left side at $0°$. Finally, leads II, aVF, and III all "look up" at the heart from below and together are called the *inferior leads* because they look at the inferior wall of the heart from the angles shown in the figure. By the same token, lead I and lead aVL are said to look at the *lateral* and *high lateral* walls of the heart, respectively.

This system of superimposing each of the limb leads on our modified compass rose is called the *hexaxial reference system.* You are urged to memorize these positions and their assigned degree values because the hexaxial reference system will become your primary tool later on when you learn to determine the electrical axis of the heart.

In the same manner as the limb leads, the V leads, placed across the precordium of the chest, "look" at the heart in the transverse plane from the positions shown in Figure 3–5. In the case of the V leads, however, we do not

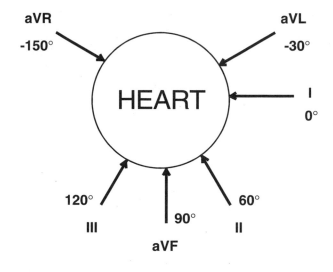

Figure 3–4
The hexaxial reference system showing the direction from which each of the limb leads "looks" at the heart in the frontal plane.

use degrees on a compass rose to assign positions. Rather, positions are assigned on the basis of actual location of the exploring electrodes as follows:

V_1—right sternal border, 4th interspace
V_2—left sternal border, 4th interspace
V_3—midway between V_2 and V_4
V_4—midclavicular line, 5th interspace
V_5—anterior axillary line, 5th interspace
V_6—midaxillary line, 5th interspace

You will learn in later chapters that, particularly in diagnosing acute myocardial infarction, small changes in the height of the R wave on the V lead recordings across the precordium can be important. Artifactual changes in R wave height can be produced merely by slightly moving the positions of the V electrodes. Therefore, when following serial ECG tracings, it is important to make certain that the V leads are placed in exactly the same positions each time an ECG is performed. To this end, it is a good idea to mark the positions on the chest wall with an indelible ink pen at the time of the first tracing so that subsequent tracings can be done with the V leads in exactly the same positions.

Figure 3–5
Position of the six V leads across the precordium.

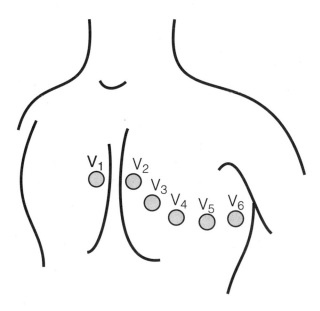

Derivation of the Normal Electrocardiogram

One of the most intimidating aspects of 12-lead electrocardiography, preventing many students from pursuing that discipline, is the thought that one will never be able to memorize what the normal electrocardiogram (ECG) looks like in all those different leads. Without realizing it, however, you have now acquired all the skills necessary to predict what the ECG will look like in each lead. Rather than memorizing, in this chapter we will figure it out together.

Important Principles

Knowledge of the following three concepts (with which you are already acquainted) is almost all that is necessary to predict the normal *morphology*, or shape, of the ECG tracing in each lead:

1. The principle that impulses coming toward an electrode produce positive deflections, whereas impulses going away from an electrode produce negative deflections
2. The positions from which the various electrodes "look" at the heart
3. The sequence, direction, and relative magnitude of the four major vectors of cardiac depolarization and repolarization

There is just one more principle of which you need to be aware, which is only a slight amplification of principle number 1. Figure 4–1 illustrates the principle that the more directly an impulse comes toward an electrode, the

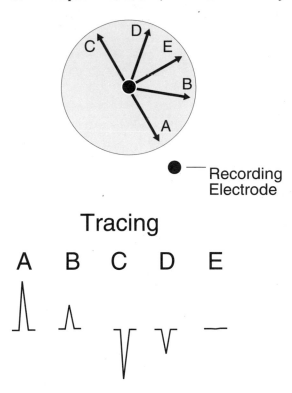

Tracing

A   B   C   D   E

Figure 4–1
Diagram of five force vectors of equal magnitude, but different directions, as recorded by a single exploring electrode.

greater will be the amplitude of the positive recorded deflection. Vector A in the illustration is coming directly toward the recording electrode and produces a very tall deflection in recording A. Vector B, on the other hand, is not coming as directly toward the electrode and therefore produces a deflection of less magnitude in recording B; that is, the positive deflection is shorter.

The same is true of impulses going away from an electrode, except the deflections in this direction are negative instead of positive. The more directly an impulse goes away from an electrode, the deeper will be the negative deflection, and the less directly an impulse goes away from an electrode, the shallower will be the negative deflection. Vector C is going directly away from the electrode and so produces a deep negative deflection. Vector D, on the other hand, is not going as directly away and so produces a deflection of lesser amplitude; that is, the deflection is less deep.

Finally, when an impulse is traveling exactly perpendicular to an electrode, that is, when it is neither coming toward nor going away from the electrode, the recorded deflection will be either isoelectric or *biphasic,* with positive and negative deflections of equal amplitude. Vector E illustrates this result.

The Normal Electrocardiogram

Now we have all the tools we need to begin to predict the appearance of a normal ECG tracing in each lead. To help us, we will superimpose our drawing of the major vectors of cardiac depolarization on the hexaxial reference system as seen in Figure 4–2.

Lead II

Let's begin with limb lead II. Lead II is located below the heart and to the left at 60°. Vector 1 represents depolarization of the atria and is coming almost directly at lead II. Since it is coming directly at lead II, we would expect a positive P wave that is quite tall and actually taller than in any other lead. That, in fact, is the case. Now you know why for so many years lead II has been used as one of the primary monitoring leads: it normally has the tallest P waves, and as a result, it is one of the leads in which it is easiest to diagnose dysrhythmias.

Vector 2 represents depolarization of the ventricular septum, so it will produce the first deflection of our QRS. It is a relatively small vector without a great deal of force. In addition, it is almost perpendicular to lead II but is, perhaps, going slightly more away from than toward lead II. So we might expect, at most, a tiny negative deflection of low amplitude as the first deflection of our QRS in lead II. Indeed, we see in our tracing that lead II often normally has a very small Q wave.

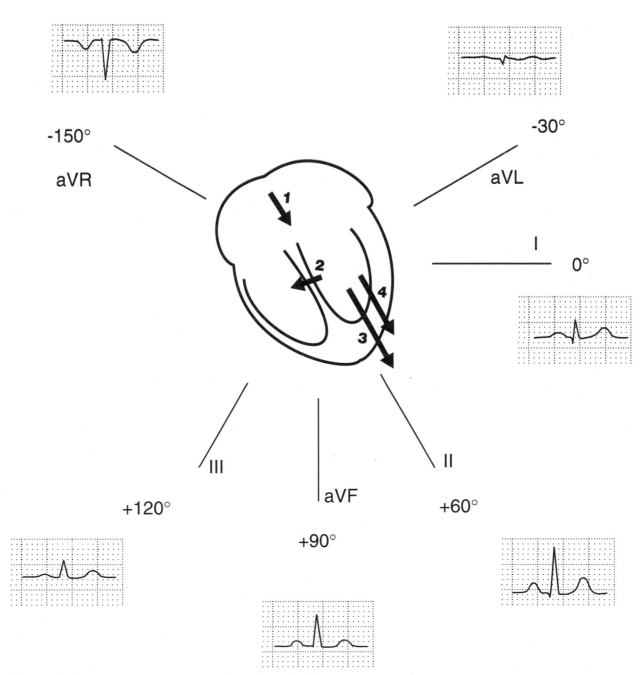

Figure 4–2. Derivation of the normal ECG in the six limb leads.

Next comes vector 3, the large summation vector of main ventricular depolarization. It is coming virtually head-on toward lead II, so we expect that the main deflection of our QRS will be positive and quite tall. And, of course, we see in our tracing that lead II has the tallest R wave of all the limb leads because vector 3 is coming more directly at lead II than at any other lead.

Finally, vector 4, representing the T wave, is also coming just about directly toward lead II, so we expect the T wave in lead II also to be positive and probably also to be the tallest of any of the limb lead T waves. Again we see in our tracings that this is, in fact, the case.

Lead aVR

Next, let's examine lead aVR because it nicely illustrates what happens when vectors are going away from a lead. Remember that lead aVR looks down on the heart from above and to the right at −150°.

Vector 1, our P wave vector, is going almost directly away from lead aVR, so we expect our P wave to be negative and quite deep.

Vector 2, the vector of our first QRS deflection, is actually coming slightly more toward than away from lead aVR. So perhaps the first deflection of our QRS will be positive, but if so, it certainly should be of very low amplitude, and in Figure 4–2, we do see a tiny R wave in lead aVR as a quite normal finding.

One can easily see, however, that a very slight counterclockwise shift in the direction of vector 2 would mean that it was going more away from lead aVR than toward it, in which case we would no longer have a small R wave. The same shift in direction, rotating the vector more toward lead II, would cause us to lose our small Q wave in lead II. Indeed, it is for this reason that the presence of both the small R wave in lead aVR and the small Q wave in lead II are normally variable.

Vector 3, our vector of main QRS deflection, is, like the P wave vector, going almost, but not quite, directly away from lead aVR. So we expect a predominantly negative S wave in lead aVR, but it should not be quite as deep as the lead II R wave is tall. This is because vector 3 is going directly toward lead II but not as directly away from lead aVR. The QRS in lead aVR will therefore not register quite as much voltage as will the QRS in lead II.

Similarly, we can expect vector 4 to produce a negative T wave in lead aVR, again of slightly less amplitude than the positive T wave in lead II.

Lead aVL

Lead aVL is the lead that is normally the most perpendicular to vector 3, the vector of main ventricular depolarization. If the direction of vector 3 is +60° and lead aVL is looking at the vector from −30°, then lead aVL is at exactly a right angle (90°) to vector 3.

Since our P wave vector is inclined at slightly less than +60°, it is going more toward than away from lead aVL, and our P wave should therefore be positive but of low amplitude.

Vector 2 is clearly traveling away from lead aVL, so a readily visible Q wave in lead aVL is not surprising.

Vector 3, at +60°, is exactly perpendicular to lead aVL, so we expect our QRS to be equally biphasic and of low amplitude.

Vector 4, also at right angles to lead aVL, may produce a practically isoelectric T wave.

Note that very minor changes, in either direction, of vectors 1, 3, or 4 could make the ECG tracing in lead aVL either predominantly positive or predominantly negative. For this reason, the P, QRS, and T waves may be normally either positive or negative in lead aVL, although they all commonly follow each other in the direction of inscription.

Lead III

Vector 1 will clearly produce a positive P wave in lead III, although not as tall as the P wave we saw in lead II.

In the case of vector 2, we now have a situation in which the direction of septal depolarization is coming toward our electrode. As a result, a small positive deflection is produced which simply contributes to the height of the R wave rather than producing a small Q wave as we saw in leads aVL and II.

Vector 3, of course, produces a predominantly positive QRS, but again the R wave is not as tall as in lead II because vector 3 is coming less directly toward lead III. As usual, the T wave simply follows the predominant direction of the QRS.

Leads I and aVF

The reader can now go through the same exercise with the two remaining leads (I and aVF) and easily derive the normal ECG pattern in each one. It is obvious that lead I will have a pattern somewhat intermediate between that of leads aVL and II and that lead aVF will have a pattern that falls between the patterns of leads II and III.

The V Leads

We can now go through a similar exercise in predicting what the normal V leads will look like. Figure 4–3 shows the position of the precordial electrodes in relation to the heart. It is important to understand that the exact position of the electrodes in relation to the heart varies from person to person and from technician to technician.

The V_1 electrode may be slightly to the right of (above) the atria over the mid-right atrium or even to the left of (below) the atrium, but it is always above the ventricles. For this reason, the P waves in lead V_1 of the normal ECG may be either negative, biphasic, or positive, but the QRS is always negative (Fig. 4–4).

In most people, lead V_1 actually looks very much like lead aVR because the main vector of ventricular depolarization is going away from both leads.

As in lead aVR, there is a small R wave in lead V_1, reflecting septal depolarization. By the same token, septal depolarization is also responsible for producing a small normal Q wave in the left precordial leads, V_5 and V_6.

Somewhere in the vicinity of leads V_2 to V_4, the electrode usually reaches the level of the midventricle. At this point, the P waves are naturally positive, and the QRS becomes biphasic because the electrode is beginning to pick up

Figure 4–3
Position of the V leads. Diagram illustrating the position of the V leads relative to the heart anteriorly. Leads V_5 and V_6 are positioned in the same interspace as V_4 (the 5th interspace) but go into the page laterally around the patient's left side. Note that the right ventricle actually lies anterior to the left ventricle, as well as to the right, and that the apex of the heart is pointed slightly to the left.

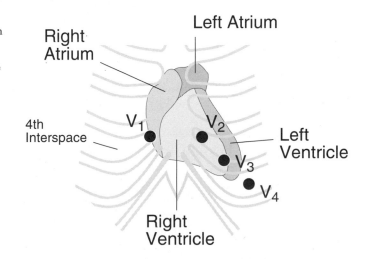

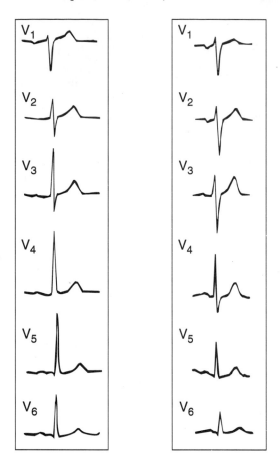

Figure 4–4
The normal V leads. The first tracing displays a transition zone in V_2; the second tracing displays transition zones in leads V_3 and V_4.

the small vectors coming toward it from endocardium to epicardium over the right ventricle as well as the vectors spreading away from it down over the left ventricle. Note in Figure 4–3 that the left ventricle actually lies posterior to the right ventricle.

The point at which the QRS becomes biphasic is called the *transition zone* because it is here that the predominant QRS deflection transitions from negative to positive. One of the results of this transition is that the R wave, normally small in lead V_1, progressively increases in height as one moves from right to left across the precordium, until the QRS is fully upright in leads V_5 and V_6. You will later learn that this normal *R wave progression* is frequently lost in anterior wall myocardial infarction.

The T wave is variable in leads V_1 and V_2 but normally becomes upright by the time one reaches the transition zone.

In summary, anything can happen with regard to P waves and T waves in leads V_1 and V_2, but they should both be upright by lead V_3. The QRS should always be predominantly negative in lead V_1, can be biphasic from leads V_2 to V_4, and should always be upright in leads V_5 and V_6.

The Layout of Three-Channel Tracings

Now that we have deduced the normal morphology of the electrocardiogram in each individual lead, we can finally put them all together in a full, normal 12-lead ECG as seen in Figure 4–5. This ECG tracing shows the usual order of lead display utilized by today's three-channel machines. All three horizontal panels are displaying the same beats, simultaneously seen in three leads. The

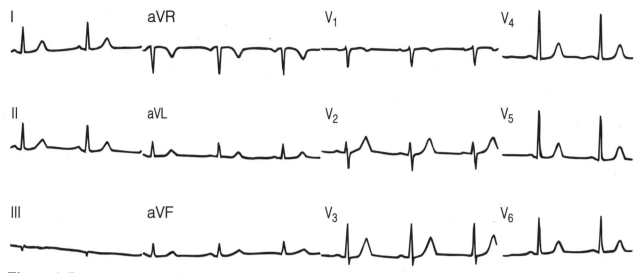

Figure 4–5. A normal 12-lead ECG. Note that in this example, both the P wave and the T wave are inverted in V_1. The transition zone occurs in V_2.

opportunity to see each beat in three leads simultaneously is especially helpful in the diagnosis of dysrhythmias.

Note that as the machine changes leads in each of the three panels, there is no pause at the time of lead change, so calipers can be used to plot intervals all the way across the tracing without interruption.

Note also that in this example (Fig. 4–5) of a normal ECG, lead III is almost equally biphasic and lead I has a slightly more positive deflection than in Figure 4–2. This means that, in this quite normal patient, all of our vectors (vectors 1 to 4) are inclined slightly more to the left than in Figure 4–2. Since lead III is almost isoelectric, vector 3 must be at about a right angle to lead III, or at about +30°. Without realizing it, you have just determined the electrical axis of this tracing, the subject of our next chapter.

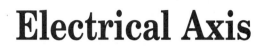

Electrical Axis

In this chapter, you will discover, happily enough, that you now have all the tools necessary to determine electrical axis, a fairly easy exercise that has the unfair reputation of being difficult.

The Definition of Electrical Axis

The term *electrical axis* normally refers to nothing more than determining the direction, or angle in degrees, in which the main vector of ventricular depolarization is pointed, that is, the direction of our old friend, vector 3. For the purpose of determining electrical axis, we therefore use the by now familiar hexaxial reference system. The precordial V leads are not used in the determination of electrical axis.

As stated earlier, in the average person, vector 3 has a direction of about 60°. Although 60° is the average, there is actually a wide range of normal, as is usually the case among human beings. Most authorities agree that the main summation vector of ventricular depolarization can quite normally point anywhere between 0° and 90°.

When the vector points further counterclockwise than 0°, we say that the tracing displays *left axis deviation* (LAD) because the vector is pointing off to the patient's left (Fig. 5–1). When the vector points further clockwise than 90°, we say that the tracing displays *right axis deviation* (RAD) because the vector is pointing off to the right. If the deviation from normal is greater than −30° or +120°, most electrocardiographers then call it *marked LAD* or *marked RAD*. Deviations of less than this are usually described as *slight*.

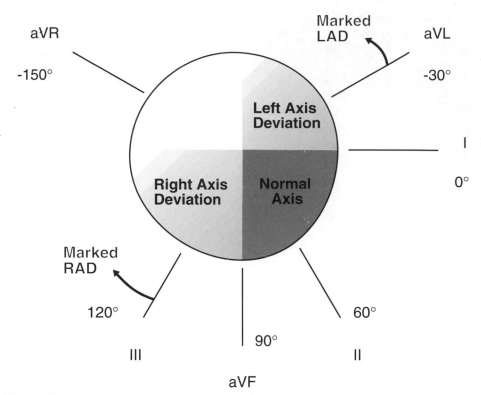

Figure 5–1. The hexaxial reference system shaded to show regions of normal axis and axis deviation.

How to Determine Electrical Axis

The Tallest R Wave

We know from previous chapters that the limb lead with the tallest R wave is going to be the lead at which vector 3 is most directly pointed. So the easiest way to roughly determine electrical axis is simply to look for the limb lead with the tallest R wave. We then know that vector 3 is pointed roughly in that direction or at least closer to that lead than to any other lead. Thus, as is illustrated in Figure 5–2A, if the tallest R wave is seen in lead II, we know that the axis is roughly +60°. If, on the other hand, the tallest R wave is seen in lead aVL, as in Figure 5–2B, we know that the axis is roughly −30°, and so on.

The Deepest S Wave

It is also easy to understand from our previous discussion of the derivation of the normal ECG that an alternate method of roughly determining axis would be to look for the lead with the deepest negative deflection, or S wave. We would then know that vector 3 was going more directly away from that lead than from any other lead. Therefore, the axis of vector 3 should be in roughly the opposite direction, or 180° from the lead with the deepest S wave. If lead aVR has the deepest S wave, then the electrical axis should be directly opposite on the hexaxial reference system, or roughly +30° (Fig. 5–2C).

Ninety Degrees from an Equally Biphasic QRS

The two methods described in the preceding paragraphs provide us with only a rough indication of the direction of the main ventricular depolarization vector. To be more accurate, we will have to refine our methods.

A third, more accurate method of determining axis is to look for a QRS that is either *equally biphasic* (that is, the positive and negative deflections are of equal amplitude) or essentially isoelectric. We know from previous discussions that when we see a lead with an equally biphasic QRS, it means that vector 3 is perpendicular to that lead.

The ECG in Figure 5–2C shows an equally biphasic QRS in lead III. So we know that our vector is perpendicular to, or 90° from, this lead. What we can't tell from looking solely at lead III, however, is whether the perpendicular vector is pointed toward the right lower quadrant or the left upper quadrant of our hexaxial reference system. To determine which quadrant, we simply look for the tallest R wave, which in this case we find in lead II. Now we can determine the axis to be approximately 90° from lead III pointed toward the right lower quadrant, or 30°.

But what if we can't find a QRS that is exactly equally biphasic? In that instance, we look for the QRS that comes closest to being equally biphasic. If it's a little more positive than negative, then we know that the vector is coming slightly more toward than away from that lead, and therefore the axis will be slightly less than 90° from our biphasic QRS. If, on the other hand, the negative deflection is of slightly greater amplitude than the positive deflection, we know that the vector is pointed slightly more away from our lead than 90°. Figure 5–2B shows a biphasic QRS in lead II that is slightly more negative than positive. Therefore, we know that the axis is actually slightly further counterclockwise from lead II than 90°, perhaps about −95°. A more refined determination would thus place the axis in Figure 5–2B at about −35°.

Midway Between the Two Equally Tallest R Waves

Obviously, not every patient is going to make it easy on us by having an electrical axis that is pointed exactly at a given lead or exactly perpendicular to a given lead. More frequently, the axis will point somewhere between two adjacent leads.

Let's say that we have a patient with an axis of 75°. That would mean that our vector was pointing exactly midway between leads II and aVF. In this instance, we could expect that instead of having one lead with the tallest R wave, we would have two leads with equally tall R waves, namely II and aVF (Fig. 5–2D). It is clear then that locating the axis midway between the two tallest R waves of equal height improves our accuracy.

Shifted Toward the Taller of the Two Tallest R Waves

But what if the two tallest R waves are not of equal height—if one is slightly taller than the other? In this instance, we need to shift our estimation of the axis slightly more toward the taller of the two R waves. For example, if our patient above had an axis of 70°, instead of 75°, then the vector would be going slightly more toward lead II than toward lead aVF, and lead II would therefore have a slightly taller R wave than lead aVF (Fig. 5–2E).

A word of caution here. This method works only when the axis is in the right lower quadrant between 0° and 90° (leads I and aVF). The reason can be seen by examining the tracing in Figure 5–2F. Note that lead aVL has the

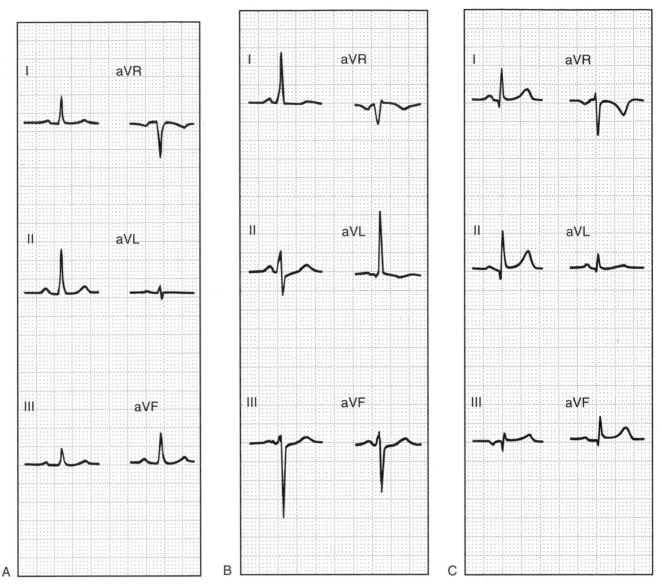

Figure 5–2. *A.* The tallest R wave is seen in lead II, placing the axis at roughly +60°. *B.* The tallest R wave is seen in lead aVL, placing the axis at roughly −30°. *C.* The deepest S wave is seen in lead aVR, placing the axis roughly directly opposite or at approximately 30°. An equally biphasic QRS in lead III places the axis perpendicular to lead III or also at approximately 30°.

Illustration continued on following page

tallest R wave, and lead I has the next tallest R wave. If we use only the method of placing the axis between the two tallest R waves and then shifting toward the taller of the two, we would estimate the axis to be about −20° or −25°. However, if we look for an isoelectric lead, we find that lead aVR is equally biphasic. That would place the axis at −60°. In this case, both leads I and aVL would be expected to be positive, with lead aVL taller than lead I because the vector is going more directly toward lead aVL than toward lead I, and indeed when we look at the tracing, we find that to be the case. Thus, when outside the right lower quadrant of the hexaxial reference system, we cannot reliably use alone the method of placing the axis between the two tallest R waves and then shifting it toward the taller of the two.

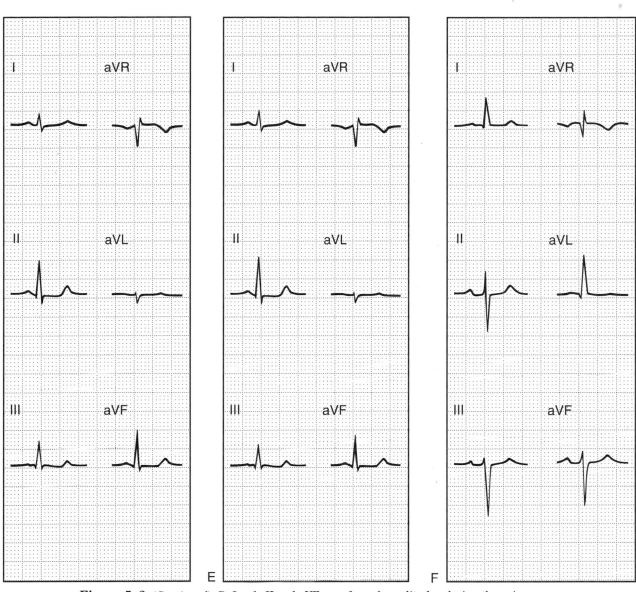

Figure 5–2. *(Continued). D.* Leads II and aVF are of equal amplitude, placing the axis midway between the two leads, or at 75°. *E.* Lead II has a slightly taller R wave than lead aVF, shifting the axis slightly more toward II, or at about 70°. *F.* Lead aVR is equally biphasic, placing the axis at −60°.

Putting It All Together

After a little practice in determining axis, you will find yourself, without consciously thinking about it, naturally using all of the above methods in a very rapid sequence to determine axis. A very quick glance for the tallest R wave establishes the general direction of the axis. Looking for an equally biphasic QRS is usually the next natural step, followed by a quick slight shifting of the axis based on whether the positive or negative deflection is the greater in our biphasic QRS. Finally, for axes within the right lower quadrant, we can shift the axis slightly more toward the taller of the two tallest R waves. With a little practice, you will find yourself capable of determining axis within 10 or 15 degrees within a matter of seconds.

The Significance of Axis Deviation

Why bother determining axis in the first place? Since the term electrical axis generally refers to the direction of the vector of main ventricular depolarization, anything that changes the determinants of the direction of ventricular depolarization can cause an axis shift.

We know from previous discussions that the factors that cause the average vector of ventricular depolarization to be at 60° include the sequence in which the various portions of ventricular muscle are activated and the normally greater muscle mass of the left ventricle, as well as, obviously, the physical position of the heart itself within the chest cavity. So anything that changes the sequence of ventricular activation, the muscle mass of either ventricle, or the position of the heart within the chest can cause axis deviation.

Before you go on, take a little time now to try to figure out, on the basis of this information, what disease processes might be expected to cause axis deviation. Then compare your list with the list at the end of this chapter. With a little thought, you may find that you have guessed quite a few of them, and you will learn why understanding is a much better method of learning than is memorizing.

You will learn also, in later chapters, that right or left axis deviation is a part of the criteria for many electrocardiographic diagnoses. Now, we will reveal some of the causes of axis deviation.

Sequences of Ventricular Activation

Common causes of a change in the sequence of ventricular activation that will result in axis deviation obviously include delays in conduction through either the right bundle branch or the left bundle branch or through one or the other of the two left hemibundles. A conduction delay or block in any one of these structures will change the sequence in which the various portions of the ventricles are activated and thus will change the direction of travel of the main vector of ventricular depolarization.

For example, if the right bundle branch is blocked, then the impulse will go down the left bundle normally, activating the left ventricle first. The only way for the right ventricle to then be depolarized is for the depolarization wave to spread across muscle from the left ventricle to the right ventricle. This produces a large vector spreading from left to right and so may cause right axis deviation (Fig. 5–3).

Changes in Ventricular Muscle Mass

You will recall that the relatively greater muscle mass of the left ventricle is one of the factors that shifted our normal vector of main ventricular depolarization slightly toward the left ventricle. This is because larger muscle masses generate greater voltages. By the same token, if we have a disease that causes right ventricular hypertrophy, such as pulmonic valve stenosis, then the enlarging muscle mass of the right ventricle will tend to shift the axis of our main vector toward the right ventricle and therefore cause right axis deviation.

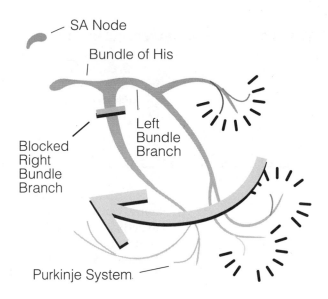

Figure 5–3
Schematic showing one of the kinds of change in sequence of activation of the ventricles that can shift electrical axis. In this example, right bundle branch block (RBBB) is present. The impulse comes down the left bundle normally, activating the left ventricle via the Purkinje system. The right bundle, however, fails to conduct the impulse, and the right ventricle is depolarized by a wave of depolarization spreading across muscle from the left ventricle to the right ventricle. This may shift the main vector of ventricular depolarization to the right, producing right axis deviation.

Physical or Mechanical Changes in the Position of the Heart

Finally, we could obviously change the direction of our main vector of ventricular depolarization by simply altering the position of the heart within the chest cavity. A simple example is the quite healthy and normal state of pregnancy. The growing uterus puts pressure on the bottom of the diaphragm, pushing the apex of the heart up to the left into a more horizontal position, thereby mechanically altering the direction of vector 3 and producing left axis deviation.

Major Causes of Left Axis Deviation

Left bundle branch block
Left anterior hemiblock
Premature ventricular contractions (PVCs) from the right ventricle
Wolff-Parkinson-White (WPW) syndrome activating the right ventricle
Left ventricular hypertrophy
Pregnancy
Ascites
Abdominal tumors
Exhalation

Major Causes of Right Axis Deviation

Right bundle branch block
Left posterior hemiblock
PVCs from the left ventricle
WPW syndrome activating the left ventricle
Right ventricular hypertrophy
Emphysema
Inhalation

A Word About Indeterminate Axis

Occasionally you will see an ECG in which all of the limb leads display an equally biphasic QRS, making determination of a single axis impossible. In such instances, you will often see the axis described as being *indeterminate* (Fig. 5–4).

Axis of P and T Waves

Although the term electrical axis in general parlance refers to the axis of main ventricular depolarization, it is obviously also possible to determine, in exactly the same fashion, the axis of the P wave or of the T wave. Although sometimes useful, determining the axes of these two waves is not usually considered a routine part of ECG interpretation.

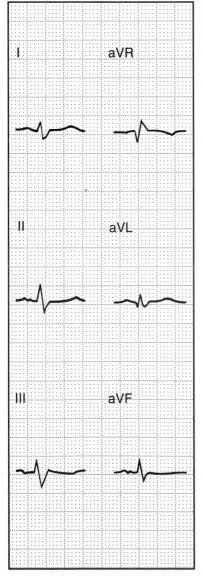

Figure 5–4
Indeterminate axis. A single axis cannot be calculated for this tracing, which shows an almost equally biphasic QRS in all leads.

▓ Practice Tracings

Figures 5–5 through 5–8 offer you some practice in your newly acquired skill of determining electrical axis. The answers may be found in the Appendix.

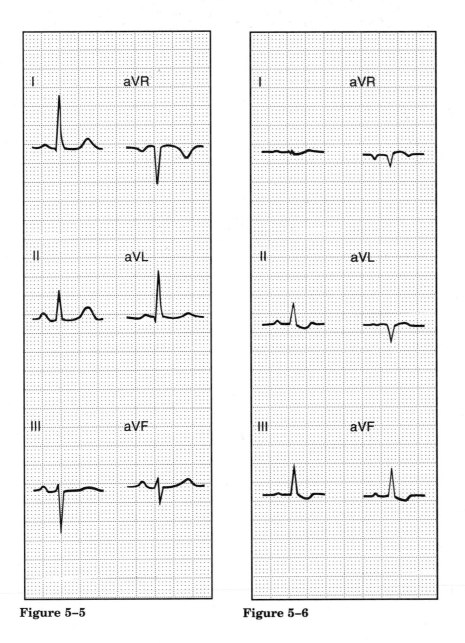

Figure 5–5

Figure 5–6

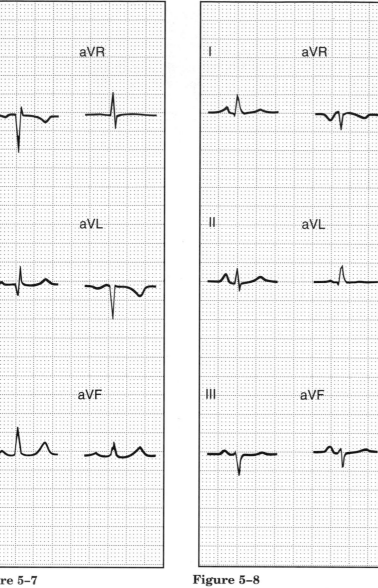

Figure 5–7   **Figure 5–8**

Intraventricular Conduction Delays: The Hemiblocks

Having just completed a study of electrical axis, we now will logically turn our attention to the so-called hemiblocks since their diagnosis depends so heavily on marked shifts in electrical axis.

Anatomy

You will recall from Chapter 1 (see Fig. 1–1) that the left bundle divides very early into a left anterosuperior fascicle and a left posteroinferior fascicle. In cross-section, one can readily see that these two fascicles run toward the *anterior* and *posterior papillary muscles,* respectively (Fig. 6–1). In reality, there is an additional third fascicle, called the *centriseptal fascicle,* that supplies the septum, but since it has little clinical bearing electrocardiographically, we will stick with the simpler clinical concept of two major divisions of the left bundle.

Failure of the Fascicles

As you might surmise, anything that can go wrong will go wrong. So, of course, we can foresee occasions when, for whatever reason, one or the other (or both) of the two fascicles will fail to work properly. Failure may include delays in repolarization, so that the impulse finds the fascicle still refractory;

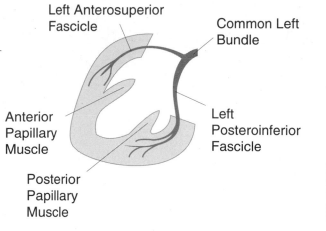

Figure 6–1
Schematic section through the left ventricle as viewed from the patient's left (posterior axillary view), showing how the anterior and posterior fascicles of the left bundle run toward their respective papillary muscles.

conduction of impulses more slowly than usual; or complete inability to conduct an impulse at all.

When either the anterosuperior or posteroinferior fascicle fails, we say that it is "blocked," and we call the failure *hemiblock*. In everday parlance, we shorten the names to *left anterior hemiblock* and *left posterior hemiblock*.

Effect of Hemiblock on Sequence of Activation—Left Anterior Hemiblock

As you know from Chapter 5, any change in the sequence of activation of the ventricles will change the axis or direction of vector 3, our main vector of ventricular depolarization. To illustrate the impact of hemiblocks, let's begin by considering left anterior hemiblock.

In left anterior hemiblock, the impulse comes down the main left bundle and the left posterior fascicle quite normally (Fig. 6–2). However, the impulse

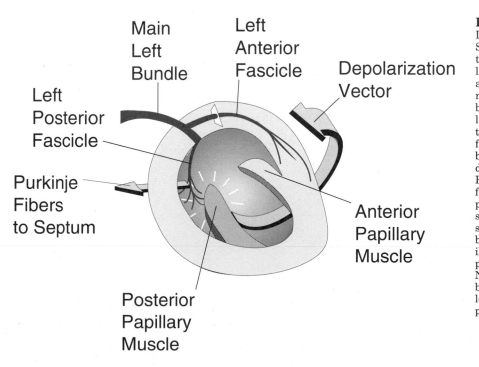

Figure 6–2
Left anterior hemiblock. Schematic frontal section through the anterior wall of the left ventricle, just anterior to the anterior papillary muscle. The right ventricle is not seen because it lies anterior to the left ventricle and is cut away. In this illustration, the anterior fascicle of the left bundle is blocked. As a result, depolarization is initiated by the Purkinje system of the posterior fascicle behind the posterior papillary muscle. A vector then spreads to the patient's left and superiorly into the region served by the anterosuperior fascicle, as illustrated by the arrow, producing left axis deviation. Note that the septum will still be depolarized normally from left to right by the intact posterior fascicle.

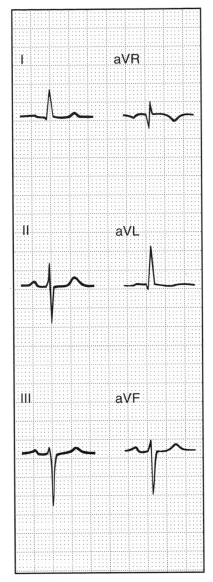

Figure 6–3
Left anterior hemiblock. Marked left axis deviation of −60⁰ is present, as is
quickly confirmed by the equally biphasic QRS in lead aVR. In addition, there is a
small R in lead III and a small Q in lead I. The QRS duration is normal.

finds the left anterior fascicle blocked. As a result, the posteroinferior section
of the ventricle is activated first. A wave of depolarization then spreads by
slow conduction from muscle fiber to muscle fiber into the portion of the ventricle normally served by the anterosuperior fascicle. The net result is a vector
spreading superiorly through the wall of the left ventricle and shifting the axis
of main ventricular depolarization counterclockwise to the left. This axis shift
is so pronounced that left anterior hemiblock usually produces marked left
axis deviation (LAD), frequently approaching −60° (Fig. 6–3). Exactly how
extreme is the LAD depends upon what the patient's normal axis was prior to
developing the hemiblock.

Although vector 3 is dramatically shifted to the left, it should be readily
apparent that septal depolarization is still occurring normally because the
posterior fascicle is still intact, and it is the posterior fascicle that predominantly supplies the septum with Purkinje fibers. Therefore, as you will note
in Figure 6–3, although the QRS in lead III is now predominantly negative,
there is still a small R wave present, reflecting normal septal depolarization.
Note that there is also still a small Q wave present in lead I, also, of course,
reflecting normal septal depolarization.

Criteria for Left Anterior Hemiblock

The diagnostic criteria, then, for isolated left anterior hemiblock include:

1. Marked left axis deviation, frequently approaching −60°
2. A small R in lead III
3. A small Q in lead I
4. Normal QRS duration

Why normal QRS duration? Although left anterior hemiblock certainly falls within the technical category of a *delay in intraventricular conduction* because it can increase QRS duration by 0.01 to 0.02 second, note in Figure 6–3 that the QRS duration is still normal. This is because, although activation of the left superior ventricle is somewhat delayed, that portion of the ventricle is a small enough area, with a short enough transit time required for the wave of muscle-to-muscle depolarization, that no significant prolongation of the QRS to 0.10 second or greater results.

Left Posterior Hemiblock

The story for left posterior hemiblock is essentially the reverse of left anterior hemiblock, as illustrated in Figure 6–4. The impulse travels down the anterior fascicle quite normally but finds the posterior fascicle blocked. As a result, the anterosuperior wall of the left ventricle is activated first, and then a slow muscle-to-muscle wave of depolarization spreads inferiorly and to the right in the direction of the posterior papillary muscle (Fig. 6–4). The net result in this instance is prominent right axis deviation (RAD) with an electrical axis that may approach +120°, again depending upon the patient's normal axis prior to developing hemiblock (Fig. 6–5).

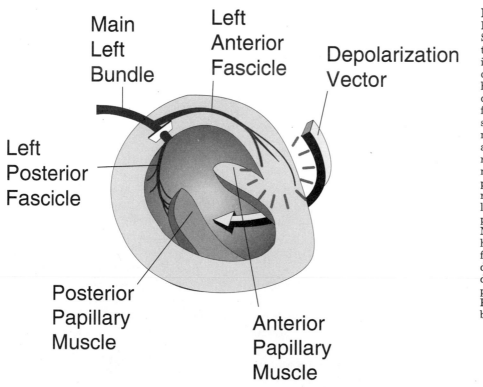

Main Left Bundle

Left Anterior Fascicle

Depolarization Vector

Left Posterior Fascicle

Posterior Papillary Muscle

Anterior Papillary Muscle

Figure 6–4
Left posterior hemiblock. Schematic frontal section through the left ventricle illustrating sequences of depolarization in left posterior hemiblock. The impulse descends the left anterior fascicle normally, then spreads by slow muscle-to-muscle conduction to the right and posteriorly toward the region of the ventricle normally served by the left posterior fascicle. The net result in the frontal plane is a left-to-right vector that produces right axis deviation. Note that in posterior hemiblock, the posterior fascicle can no longer depolarize the septum. Septal depolarization therefore takes place from right to left via Purkinje fibers from the right bundle branch (not pictured).

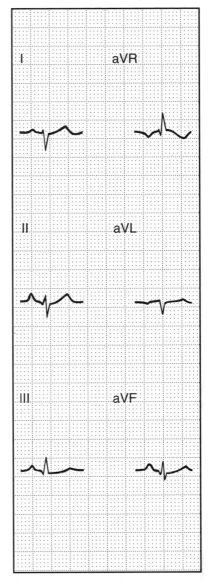

Figure 6–5
Left posterior hemiblock. Marked right axis deviation of 170⁰ is present, along with a small R in lead I and a small Q in lead III.

This time, however, since the Purkinje fibers that supply the septum are a part of the posterior fascicle and are therefore blocked, septal depolarization no longer occurs from left to right. Instead, the septum is now depolarized by the right bundle, and the result is a right-to-left vector across the septum. Thus, with left posterior hemiblock, we now see in Figure 6–5 a small Q in lead III and a small R in lead I—just the opposite of what we see with left anterior hemiblock. As before, QRS duration remains normal.

Criteria for Left Posterior Hemiblock

In summary, then, the criteria for isolated left posterior hemiblock are:

1. Right axis deviation, often approaching +120°
2. Small Q in lead III
3. Small R in lead I
4. Normal QRS duration

Confusion of Left Anterior Hemiblock With Inferior Wall Myocardial Infarction

You will learn in Chapter 9 that one of the hallmarks of acute myocardial infarction is the development of Q waves. In inferior wall myocardial infarction, very deep Q waves can develop in the leads that look at the inferior wall of the heart, that is, in leads II, III, and aVF (Fig. 6–6).

Because left anterior hemiblock produces deep S waves in leads II, III, and aVF, these S waves can sometimes be mistaken for the Q waves of inferior myocardial infarction if the ECG reader does not notice the small R wave in front of the S wave (Fig. 6–7).

In inferior wall myocardial infarction, the development of the Q wave in leads II, III, and aVF eliminates the small R wave in lead III that is present in left anterior hemiblock. Thus, the presence or absence of the small R in lead III is important in helping to distinguish an inferior wall myocardial infarction

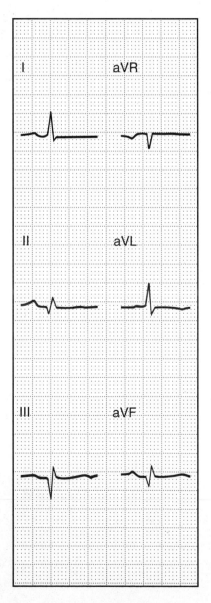

Figure 6–6
Old inferior wall myocardial infarction with Q waves in leads II, III, and aVF and with an axis of approximately -5^0.

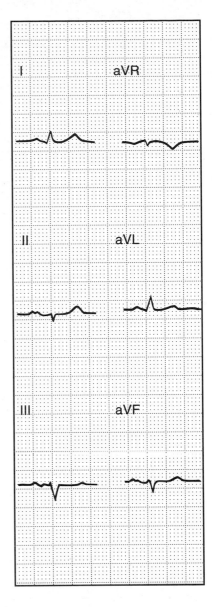

Figure 6–7
Left anterior hemiblock with deep S waves in the inferior wall (leads II, III, and aVF), which can be mistaken for old inferior myocardial infarction (MI) if the reader does not notice that there are actually tiny initial R waves present in leads III and aVF and not Q waves. In addition, the left axis deviation (LAD) is more extreme at about −50°.

from left anterior hemiblock and, for that reason, is a part of the criteria necessary to define left anterior hemiblock. This concept will become clearer after your study of myocardial infarction in Chapter 9.

In addition, note in Figure 6–6 that the presence of Q waves in inferior wall myocardial infarction alone does not usually produce the extreme LAD seen with left anterior hemiblock.

Block of Both Fascicles

I mentioned at the beginning of this chapter that it is quite possible for both the left anterior and posterior fascicles to fail to conduct an impulse. In this instance, of course, we essentially have failure of the entire left bundle, producing *left bundle branch block,* one of the subjects of our next chapter. Combinations of right bundle branch block and one or the other of the hemiblocks will also be discussed in Chapter 7.

Practice Tracings

Figures 6–8 through 6–11 offer you some practice in identifying hemiblocks. The answers may be found in the appendix.

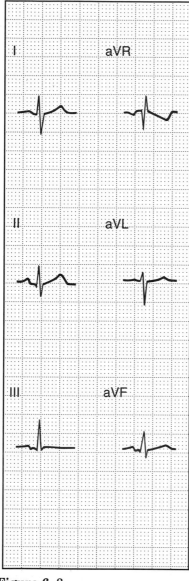

Figure 6–8

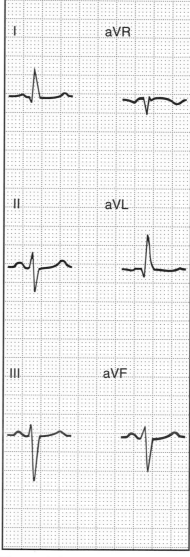

Figure 6–9

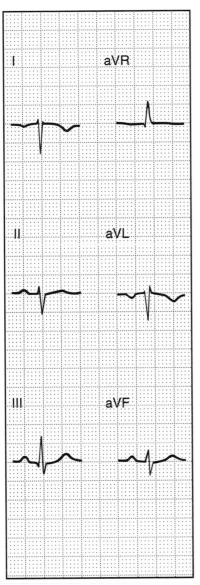

Figure 6–10

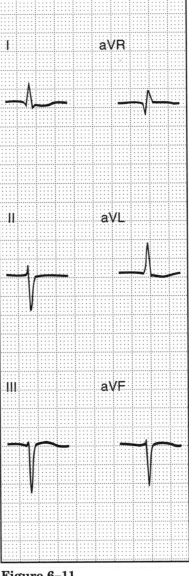

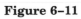

Figure 6–11

CHAPTER 7

Intraventricular Conduction Delays: The Bundle Branch Blocks

In Chapter 6, I examined delays in intraventricular conduction that do not prolong the duration of the QRS—namely, the hemiblocks. In Chapter 7, I will examine more severe intraventricular conduction delays that do result in QRS prolongation—the bundle branch blocks.

Anatomy and Pathophysiology

By now you are familiar with the specialized conduction system of the heart. *Bundle branch block* (BBB) is the pattern produced when either the right bundle or the entire left bundle (both fascicles) fails to conduct an impulse normally.

As you will recall from Chapter 6, there are essentially three mechanisms for failure of a portion of the conduction system to conduct impulses normally:

1. Delays in repolarization so that the impulse finds a portion of the conduction system still refractory
2. Reduction in the normal speed of conduction
3. Complete inability to conduct an impulse

Complete Bundle Branch Block

The bundle branch blocks are divided into two categories of severity—*complete* and *incomplete*. In complete BBB, there is total failure of the affected bundle branch to conduct an impulse. The ventricle on the side of the failed bundle branch must be depolarized by the spread of a wave of

47

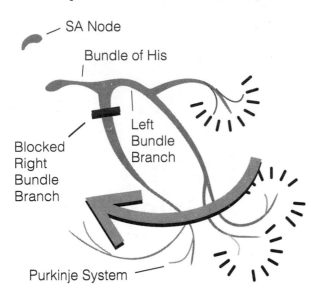

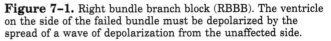

SA Node

Bundle of His

Blocked Right Bundle Branch

Left Bundle Branch

Purkinje System

Figure 7-1. Right bundle branch block (RBBB). The ventricle on the side of the failed bundle must be depolarized by the spread of a wave of depolarization from the unaffected side.

depolarization through ventricular muscle from the unaffected side (Fig. 7–1). Obviously, this activation of the affected ventricle by muscle-to-muscle conduction is a much slower process than is rapid activation through the Purkinje fibers of a normally functioning bundle branch. In addition, there is a lot of ground to cover—essentially an entire ventricle. The result is that, in complete BBB, the QRS duration is prolonged to at least 0.12 second or greater.

Incomplete Bundle Branch Block

Sometimes the blocked bundle branch is not totally blocked but merely conducts the impulse more slowly than usual. This delays depolarization of the affected ventricle long enough so that there is enough time for a wave of depolarization to begin spreading over muscle across from the unaffected side. In the meantime, the impulse also finally travels down the partially blocked bundle branch and reaches the Purkinje fibers on the affected side. The result is that part of the muscle on the affected side is activated by the conduction system and part by the slow wave of depolarization spreading over muscle from the unaffected side (Fig. 7–2). This produces a QRS that is not quite as wide as in complete BBB but is wider than normal. In other words, QRS duration in incomplete BBB is between 0.10 and 0.12 second.

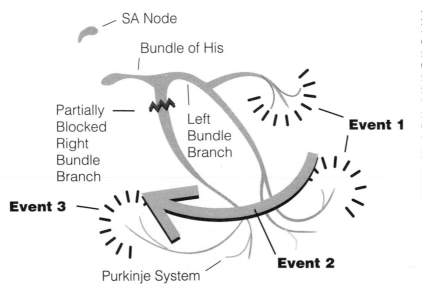

SA Node

Bundle of His

Partially Blocked Right Bundle Branch

Left Bundle Branch

Event 1

Event 2

Event 3

Purkinje System

Figure 7-2
Incomplete RBBB. The impulse comes down the left bundle normally, initiating normal depolarization of the left bundle (Event 1). Next, a slow vector of muscle-to-muscle depolarization begins to spread into the right ventricle (Event 2). Finally, the delayed impulse coming down the right bundle reaches the Purkinje fibers (Event 3). The net result is that the right ventricle is depolarized by the slow vector spreading from the left ventricle as well as by the delayed impulse coming down the right bundle. This produces a QRS that is intermediate in duration, that is, between 0.10 and 0.12 second.

Looking for Bundle Branch Blocks in the V Leads

Although the QRS is prolonged in all leads in BBB, you will see very shortly that particularly characteristic patterns are produced in the precordial leads that make it very easy to distinguish right bundle branch block (RBBB) from left bundle branch block (LBBB). For this reason, most of our discussion will concern the impact of BBB on the V leads.

Of course, there is also reason to examine the limb leads in BBB, primarily to determine electrical axis. You will learn that either right axis deviation or left axis deviation can be seen with both RBBB and LBBB and that these axis shifts do have some significance.

Complete Right Bundle Branch Block

Now, let's look at some specifics. You will note in Figure 7–3 that RBBB reverses the normal pattern of a predominantly negative QRS in lead V_1. Instead, we see an upright QRS with an RSR'. Now, let's see if we can figure out what produces this pattern. In RBBB, the impulse goes down the left bundle quite normally and activates the septum and then the left ventricle. Since the septum is depolarized normally, we can expect our initial QRS deflection to be quite normal and to produce an initial R wave in lead V_1 and a normal initial Q wave in leads V_5 and V_6.

Next, we see the beginning of an S wave in lead V_1 and an R wave in lead V_6. This reflects normal depolarization of the left ventricle. However, at this point (which is actually quite late in the QRS), our wave of depolarization in the left ventricle begins to slowly travel across muscle into the right ventricle and therefore toward lead V_1. This produces a second positive deflection in lead V_1 (the R') and a late S wave in leads V_5 and V_6. Note that the slowness of this process is reflected by the fact that the R' in lead V_1 and the S wave in leads V_5 and V_6 are quite wide and account for the increase in our QRS duration to 0.12 second or greater.

We can summarize the pattern of RBBB, then, by saying that it produces an RSR' (an upright M-shaped pattern) on the right side in lead V_1 and a prominent, wide S on the left side in leads V_5 and V_6. You will soon see that LBBB produces a very similar pattern in reverse.

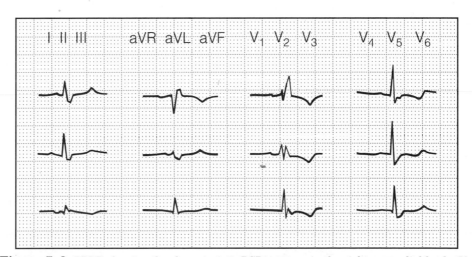

Figure 7–3. RBBB showing the characteristic RSR' pattern in the right precordial leads (V_1 and V_2) and a prominent wide S wave in the lateral precordial leads (V_5 and V_6).

Complete Left Bundle Branch Block

In Figure 7–4, you will see the pattern of LBBB and will note that, indeed, it is the reverse (although not a mirror image) of RBBB, in the sense that it produces an upright M-shaped pattern (this time on the left in leads V_5 and V_6) and a deep, negative QS on the right in leads V_1 and V_2.

In LBBB, the impulse, of course, finds the left bundle blocked and goes down the right bundle. The septum, as usual, is the first part of the ventricles to be activated, but since the left bundle is blocked, the septum is now activated by Purkinje fibers from the right bundle, producing a right-to-left vector across the septum. Thus, the first deflection of our QRS will be negative in lead V_1 and positive in lead V_6. Our normal initial R in lead V_1 becomes a Q, and our normal initial Q in lead V_6 becomes an R.

Next, the right ventricle is activated but usually does not produce an R wave in lead V_1, possibly for two reasons. The first is that the vector of right ventricular depolarization traveling from endocardium to epicardium toward lead V_1 is partially counterbalanced by the continuing right-to-left vector in the opposite direction through the septum with its greater muscle mass. The second explanation is that upon normal activation of the right ventricle, a large slow vector immediately begins to spread into the larger mass of the left ventricle, across muscle from right to left, also helping to counterbalance what would usually be our normal small R wave in lead V_1.

Nevertheless, it is worthwhile to note that occasionally the right ventricular forces spreading from endocardium to epicardium are still strong enough in LBBB to produce a tiny R wave in leads V_1 and V_2 (Fig. 7–5).

Finally, the right ventricle finishes depolarizing before the slow wave of depolarization has finished spreading from right to left across the left ventricle. This leaves the vector spreading through the left ventricle unopposed and completes the wide, deep QS that we see in lead V_1 in LBBB.

While producing a deep QS in lead V_1, the same right-to-left forces are producing a wide positive deflection in leads V_5 and V_6. Usually the QRS in the left precordial leads (V_5 and V_6) is *monophasic,* as seen in Figure 7–6, meaning that it goes in only one direction (in this case upward without a negative deflection). However, sometimes the right ventricular forces will be strong enough to produce a small S in the middle of the QRS followed by an R', thus again producing an M-shaped pattern on the left as in Figure 7–4.

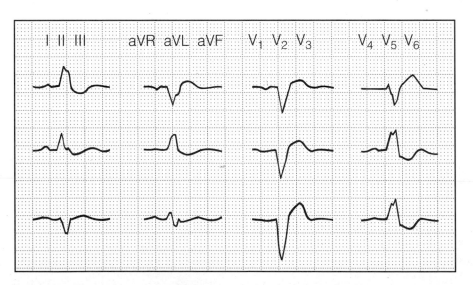

Figure 7–4
Left bundle branch block (LBBB) showing a deep QS wave in the right precordial leads (V_1 and V_2) and the typical RSR' in the left precordial leads.

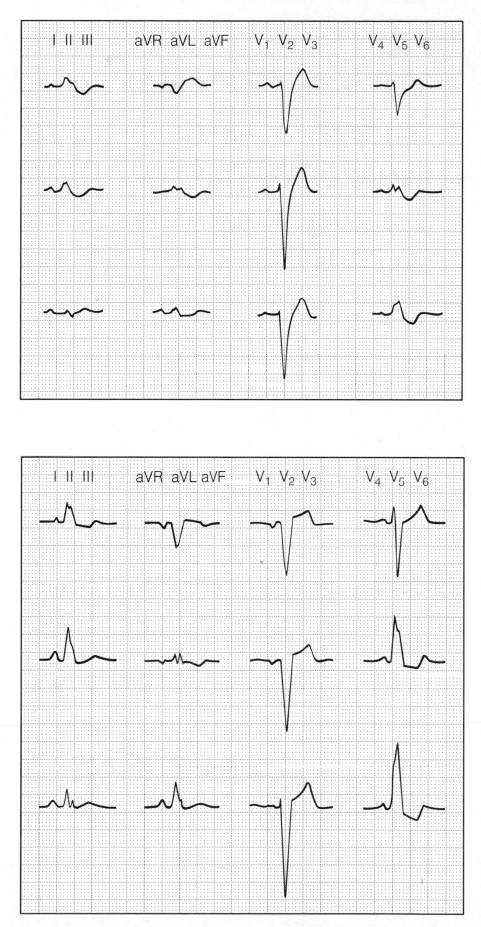

Figure 7–5
LBBB with small R waves in leads V_1 and V_2.

Figure 7–6
LBBB showing a monophasic QRS in leads V_5 and V_6 without the characteristic RSR′ pattern.

Bundle Branch Blocks, ST Segments, and T Waves

You will note that in all of the examples of BBB you have seen so far, the ST segments and T waves appear abnormal. Along with the abnormalities of depolarization in BBB come abnormalities of repolarization. Thus, it is characteristic of BBB that the T waves are usually inscribed in the opposite direction from the terminal portion of the QRS. This is because, as you learned earlier, it is the terminal portion of the QRS that reflects the large, slow, abnormal vector of muscle-to-muscle depolarization that is characteristic of BBB.

Note also that the ST segments are typically slurred into the inverted T waves. These ST and T wave changes are called *secondary changes* because they occur as the result of the intraventricular conduction delay rather than as a primary reflection of some other myocardial abnormality.

Summary of Findings in Bundle Branch Block

Figure 7–7 compares typical RBBB with LBBB. Note that RBBB displays the upright "M" on the right side of the precordial leads (V_1), and LBBB displays the upright "M" on the left side. Thus, if you simply remember right on the right and left on the left, you can easily distinguish between the two. Note also that the two are very easy to distinguish in lead V_1 alone. RBBB in lead V_1 is upright and M-shaped, and LBBB in lead V_1 is quite the opposite with a deep QS.

Incomplete Bundle Branch Block and Nonspecific Intraventricular Conduction Delays

Figure 7–8 shows a tracing with an RSR′ in lead V_2 typical of RBBB but with a narrower QRS duration of 0.10 second or greater and less than 0.12 second. You will also note that in this tracing, the QRSs are less bizarre, and there are fewer secondary ST and T wave changes. This tracing falls into the category of incomplete RBBB, referred to earlier.

The usual pattern of complete LBBB is altered in similar ways in incomplete LBBB (Fig. 7–9). These findings reflect delay in conduction of the impulse by the affected bundle branch, rather than total failure.

Not infrequently, one sees a tracing with QRS prolongation of 0.10 second or greater but without a pattern typical of either RBBB or LBBB. Electrocardiographers frequently describe such tracings as showing an intraventricular conduction delay that is *nonspecific* (Fig. 7–10).

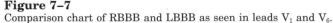

Figure 7–7
Comparison chart of RBBB and LBBB as seen in leads V_1 and V_6.

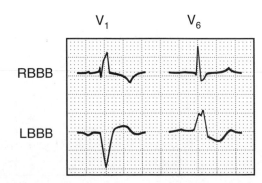

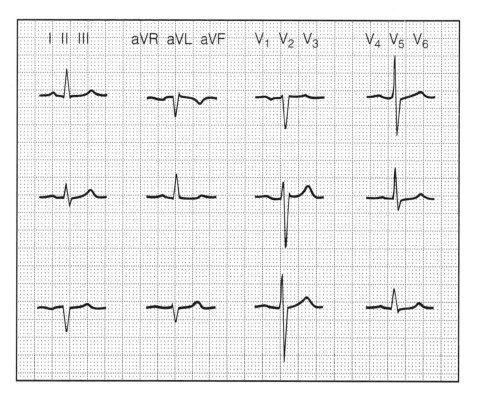

Figure 7-8
Incomplete RBBB displaying an RSR' in lead V₂ and mild QRS prolongation (QRS duration of 0.104 second but less than the 0.12 second required for complete bundle branch block). Note that few secondary ST segment and T wave changes are present.

Intermittent Bundle Branch Block and Supraventricular Aberrancy

If one of the bundle branches repolarizes slightly more slowly than the other, it would be possible to find a heart rate that would be slow enough to allow one bundle branch adequate time for repolarization, but too fast to allow the other bundle branch adequate time for repolarization. Such a circumstance produces what is called a *rate-dependent BBB*. As soon as the R-to-R intervals become shorter than the time required for repolarization of the slower of the

Figure 7-9
Incomplete LBBB showing a QRS duration of 0.116 second with either no R wave or tiny R waves in the right precordial leads (poor R wave progression) and a deep S wave. The QRS is upright on the left with only mild secondary ST segment and T wave changes.

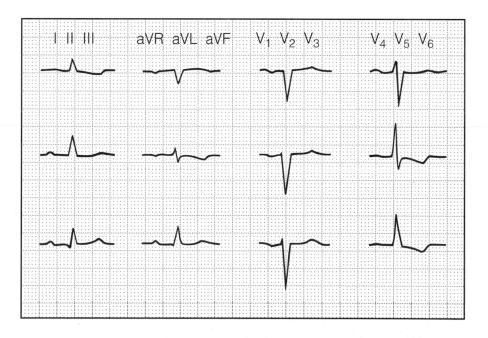

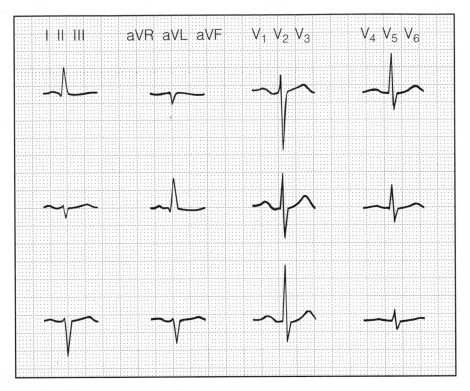

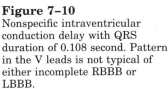

Figure 7–10
Nonspecific intraventricular conduction delay with QRS duration of 0.108 second. Pattern in the V leads is not typical of either incomplete RBBB or LBBB.

two bundle branches, the patient's tracing switches from normal conduction to a BBB pattern, as seen in Figure 7–11.

Conversely, when the patient's heart rate slows enough to allow both bundle branches adequate time for repolarization, the tracing will switch back to a pattern of normal conduction with a narrow QRS. For example, if the right bundle branch requires 600 milliseconds to repolarize, as soon as the R-to-R interval becomes shorter than 600 ms, an RBBB pattern will appear. When the R-to-R interval becomes greater than 600 ms, the RBBB pattern will disappear.

The above example is actually quite practical because in most of us it is the right bundle branch that is the slowest to repolarize. Thus, most patients who display a rate-dependent BBB develop an RBBB pattern when their rate becomes too fast.

It is exactly the same phenomenon that produces aberrant conduction of premature supraventricular beats. If, for instance, the impulse of a premature atrial contraction (PAC) reaches the bundle branches in the patient sample mentioned above in less than the 600 milliseconds required for repolarization, it will find the right bundle still refractory, and the PAC will be aberrantly conducted with an RBBB pattern (Fig. 7–12).

Thus, when it is difficult to determine whether an aberrantly conducted beat is a supraventricular beat with aberrancy or a premature ventricular

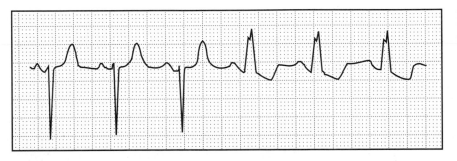

Figure 7–11
Rate-dependent bundle branch block. This patient switches conduction to an RBBB pattern when his rate reaches approximately 85.

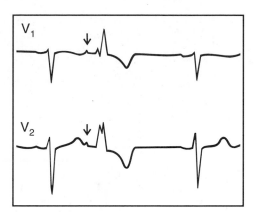

Figure 7–12
An aberrantly conducted premature atrial contraction (PAC), as seen in leads V_1 and V_2, which finds the right bundle branch still refractory and thus produces an RBBB pattern. The PAC is marked with an arrow.

contraction, the presence of an RBBB pattern makes it slightly more likely to be supraventricular since in most of us the right bundle repolarizes slightly more slowly than the left.

Relationship of Bundle Branch Block Patterns to Premature Ventricular Contractions and Paced Beats

Now that you understand why the QRS is prolonged to 0.12 second or greater in BBB, you can also understand why PVCs are always 0.12 second or greater. It is, again, because the ventricles are being activated by the slow process of muscle-to-muscle conduction rather than being rapidly depolarized through the Purkinje system.

You can also now understand that we can frequently determine the general location from which a PVC is arising by looking at its pattern in the precordial leads. A PVC arising in the left ventricle will produce a vector slowly spreading to the right ventricle and will therefore produce a pattern similar to the pattern of an RBBB (Fig. 7–13).

On the other hand, a wave of depolarization arising from a PVC in the right ventricle will slowly spread toward the left ventricle, simulating the pattern of an LBBB (Fig. 7–14).

Exactly the same phenomenon occurs when a pacemaker fires from the apex of the right ventricle. Electrocardiographically, it produces a similar pattern to that of a PVC arising from the right ventricle. Pacemakers that are properly placed in the right ventricle therefore produce an LBBB pattern (Fig. 7–15).

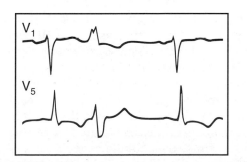

Figure 7–13. Premature ventricular contraction (PVC) arising from the left ventricle, producing an RBBB pattern.

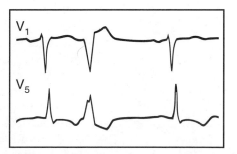

Figure 7–14. PVC arising from the right ventricle, producing an LBBB pattern.

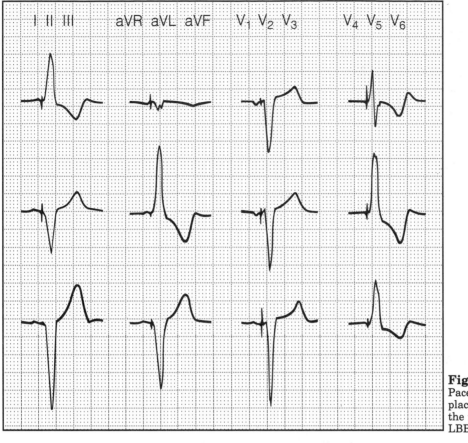

I II III   aVR aVL aVF   V₁ V₂ V₃   V₄ V₅ V₆

Figure 7–15
Paced beats from a pacemaker placed, as usual, in the apex of the right ventricle, producing an LBBB pattern.

Bifascicular and Trifascicular Block

Now that you have completed study of both the hemiblocks and the bundle branch blocks, it may have occurred to you that there might be situations in which there could be combinations of bundle block and hemiblock. Indeed, this is the case.

If we consider that there are normally three major final or distal routes for conduction of an impulse to the ventricles (the right bundle branch and the two left bundle fascicles), we can easily envision that there could be block present in two of the three or in all three pathways (fascicles).

Figure 7–16 shows a tracing with RBBB but also with extreme left axis deviation, a small Q in lead I, and a small R in lead III. This patient has both RBBB and left anterior hemiblock (LAH).

Figure 7–17 shows a tracing with typical RBBB in the precordial leads but, in this case, with extreme right axis deviation with a small R in lead I and a small Q in lead III. This represents the combination of RBBB and left posterior hemiblock (LPH). In actuality, this is the most common presentation of LPH. Isolated LPH without accompanying RBBB is very rare.

Thus, both tracings display a block of two of the three pathways, or fascicles, for impulse conduction to the ventricles, and both fall into the category of what some people call *bifascicular block*. Notice, however, that both tracings have a normal PR interval, which indicates that the impulse is getting down the remaining functioning fascicle on time. Left bundle branch block alone is also considered to be an example of bifascicular block because both the anterior and posterior left fascicles are blocked.

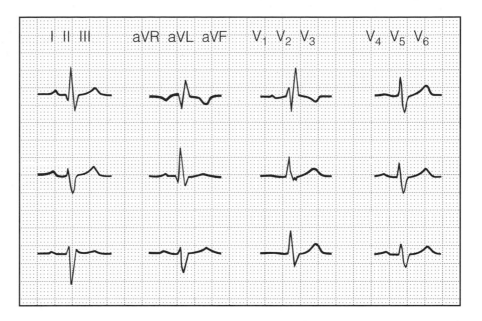

Figure 7–16
RBBB and left anterior hemiblock. Tracing displays RBBB with extreme left axis deviation (−55°), a small Q in lead I, and a small R in lead III.

As you undoubtedly have surmised by now, the term *trifascicular block* indicates either partial or complete block in all three major fascicles. Obviously, if all three fascicles are completely blocked, no impulse will reach the ventricles and, in such instances, complete atrioventricular (AV) block (third-degree block) will be present.

On the other hand, if two of the three fascicles are completely blocked but the remaining fascicle is only partially blocked, or if there is a delay in the AV node, then we could expect to see any of our examples of bifascicular block and, in addition, a prolonged PR interval (first-degree block). Thus, if Figure 7–16 showed a PR interval of 0.20 second or greater, in addition to RBBB and LAH, we would have an example of trifascicular block. Complete LBBB with a prolonged PR interval would also be an example of trifascicular block because there would be delay in the impulse coming down the remaining functioning right bundle branch.

Figure 7–17
RBBB and left posterior hemiblock. Tracing displays RBBB with extreme right axis deviation (+175°), a small R in lead I, and a very small Q in lead III.

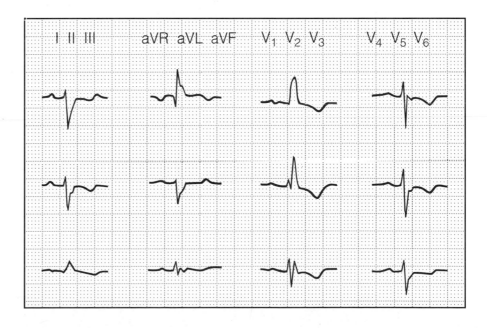

In summary, then, trifascicular block is present whenever we see a bifascicular block in addition to first-degree or higher AV block, as summarized below.

Bifascicular Block

RBBB with LAH
RBBB with LPH
LBBB

Trifascicular Block

RBBB, LAH, and first-degree or higher AV block
RBBB, LPH, and first-degree or higher AV block
LBBB and first-degree or higher AV block
Complete (third-degree) AV block

▦ Practice Tracings

Figures 7–18 through 7–21 offer you some practice in interpreting the bundle branch blocks. The answers may be found in the Appendix.

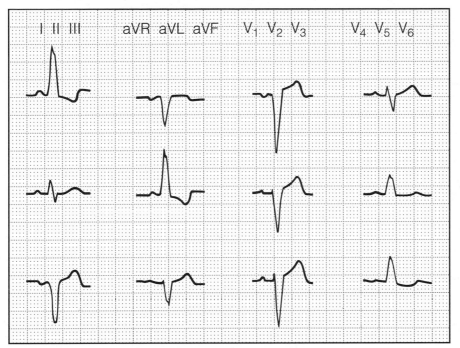

Figure 7–18

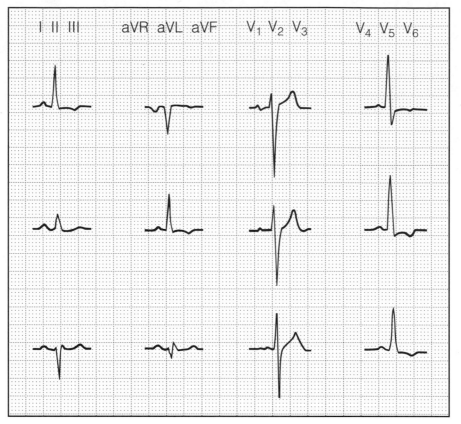

Figure 7–19

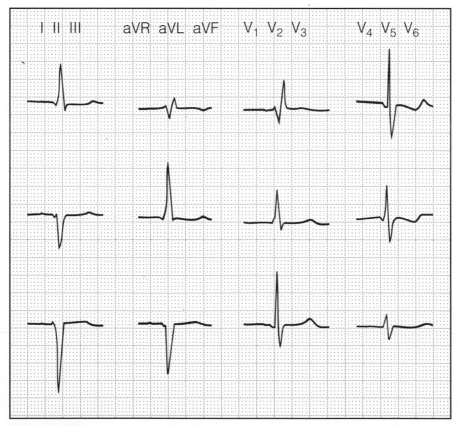

Figure 7–20

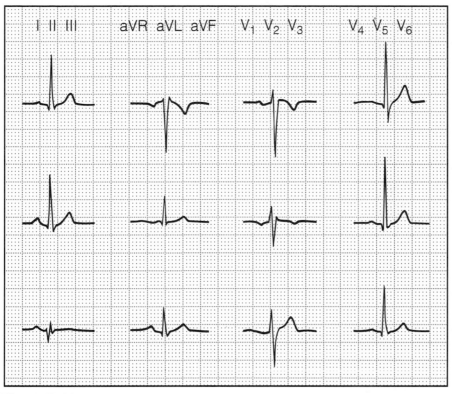

Figure 7-21

8

Chamber Enlargement

In this chapter we will examine the changes elicited in the ECG by muscular hypertrophy of the ventricles.

Pathophysiology

Like any muscle, when called upon to work harder than is normally required, cardiac muscle will enlarge, or *hypertrophy*. The cause is typically either an increased resistance to outflow of blood from the chamber (as in stenosis of a valve or hypertension) or the requirement to handle increased volumes of blood (as in regurgitation of blood across an incompletely closed valve or as in many forms of congenital heart disease).

The nature of the increased work is frequently that of generating higher pressures within the chamber during systole. In addition, diastolic pressures are frequently elevated because of either a diminished ejection fraction (the percentage of blood ejected from the chamber with each squeeze) or increased diastolic volumes of blood (as in regurgitation).

The result is increased muscle mass of the affected chamber.

Force Vectors in Chamber Enlargement

Many of the ECG changes caused by hypertrophy of cardiac muscle can be deduced from your knowledge of the behavior of cardiac force vectors. You already know, for example, that the larger the muscle mass, the larger the force vector and therefore the greater the voltage in the ECG. We could surmise then that the QRS would show excessive voltage in ventricular hypertrophy.

In addition, you know that changes in the wall thickness of either the right ventricle or the left ventricle could change the direction of the vector of main ventricular depolarization. We could also surmise then that we could see a change in electrical axis with ventricular hypertrophy.

Finally, it is logical that the greater the muscle mass, the longer it takes for a wave of depolarization to traverse that muscle mass. So, we could again surmise that it would be possible to see slightly increased QRS duration in the presence of ventricular hypertrophy.

Of course, all of these features may be seen in ventricular hypertrophy.

Left Ventricular Hypertrophy

In left ventricular hypertrophy (LVH), the muscle mass of the left ventricle enlarges. This tilts the main vector of ventricular depolarization more toward the left ventricle and, of course, increases its magnitude. As a result, the S wave in lead V_1 becomes deeper, and the R wave in the lateral precordial leads (V_5 and V_6) becomes taller. It follows that the electrical axis may be shifted more toward the left, often, but not always, resulting in left axis deviation. Increased amplitude of the R wave is also therefore frequently seen in limb lead I or aVL.

Figure 8–1 shows the ECG of a 38-year-old white male with longstanding severe hypertension. Note that the S wave in lead V_1 is 31 mm deep, and the R wave in lead V_4 is 30 mm tall.

Many different voltage criteria for LVH have been proposed, but most electrocardiographers would agree that LVH is likely if the S wave in leads V_1 or V_2 or the R wave in leads V_5 or V_6 reaches 30 mm or more in magnitude. As always, there are many normal variants among humans. Individuals with thin chest walls (children in particular) and individuals who are the size of professional basketball players may have greater than 30 mm of QRS voltage in the absence of LVH.

QRS duration in LVH is usually only mildly increased, if at all, toward the upper limits of normal, between 0.09 and 0.10 second. This is because, although the wall of the ventricle is thicker, the wall is still being depolarized by impulses spreading through the rather rapidly conducting Purkinje system. The function of the Purkinje system is the greater determining factor in QRS duration. Figure 8–1 shows a QRS duration of 0.09 second.

Certain changes in the ST and T waves can also develop in LVH, usually most prominently in the lateral precordial leads (V_5 and V_6) but also in those limb leads toward which the main vector of depolarization is traveling (electrical axis). As hypertrophy progresses, downsloping ST depression and T wave inversion can occur, which, in the fully developed pattern, is called *left ventricu-*

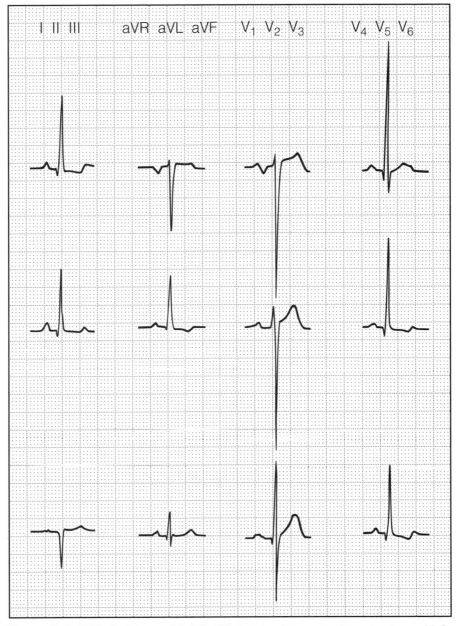

Figure 8–1. ECG of a 38-year-old male with longstanding severe hypertension and left ventricular hypertrophy (LVH). Note the deep S wave in leads V_1 and V_2, the tall R wave in lead V_4 (exceeding 30 mm), a QRS duration at the upper limits of normal at .09 second, and an axis shifted toward the left at +18°.

lar strain. Figure 8–2 shows a fully developed strain pattern in which the ST depression is typically *upwardly convex* with a gentle transition into an inverted T wave. These ST and T wave changes are called *secondary* because they are secondary to the LVH rather than being a direct reflection of another primary myocardial abnormality. As you will learn later, the strain pattern can be confused with ST and T wave changes caused by myocardial ischemia, myocardial infarction, and other miscellaneous conditions, such as digitalis effect.

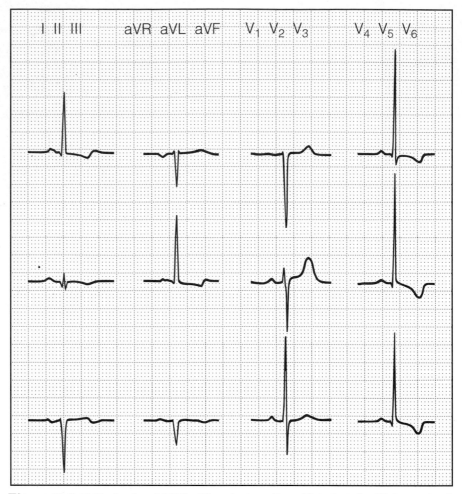

Figure 8–2. Fully developed LVH with a strain pattern. Note that the ST depression is upwardly convex and gently transitions to an inverted T. This patient also meets voltage criteria of 30 mm in lead V_5 and left axis deviation (LAD) with an axis of $-27°$.

Summary of Criteria for LVH

None of the above criteria, taken alone, is a reliable indicator for LVH. You will often see ECG interpretations that read something like "LVH by voltage criteria alone." This is the electrocardiographer's way of saying that although voltage criteria are present for LVH, there are no other criteria present, and he cannot guarantee that LVH really exists in this patient.

Conversely, LVH may be present without all of the electrocardiographic criteria being met. In other words, the criteria have both *low specificity* and *low sensitivity* for LVH. The more criteria present, therefore, the more likely it is that LVH is present. The following is a summary of things to look for in trying to diagnose LVH by ECG:

1. S wave in lead V_1 or V_2 or R wave in lead V_5 or V_6 of 30 mm or greater
2. Left axis deviation
3. QRS duration at the upper limit of normal
4. Shift in the ST segment or T wave (strain pattern) in leads V_5 and V_6

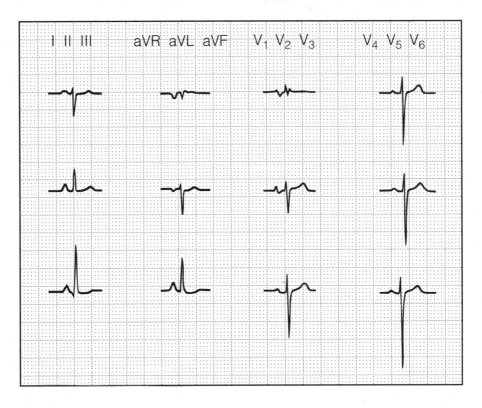

Figure 8–3
Right ventricular hypertrophy
(RVH) with a tall R wave in the
right-sided precordial leads and
a deep S in the left-sided
precordial leads.

Right Ventricular Hypertrophy

We turn our attention now to the right ventricle, where all of the same principles apply. A major difference, however, is that the right ventricle has a much smaller muscle mass to begin with than has the left ventricle. Therefore, in order for the right ventricle to surpass the left ventricle in size and shift our vectors substantially to the right, it has to hypertrophy rather massively. This means that, again, our ECG criteria are not going to be very sensitive indicators of early right ventricular hypertrophy (RVH). This also accounts for the fact that full-blown RVH on an ECG is relatively rare, especially in adults.

In RVH, as the right ventricular muscle mass increases, the direction of our main vector of ventricular depolarization naturally shifts progressively toward the right. This produces a taller than normal R wave in the right-side precordial leads (V_1 and V_2). As you would guess, this also produces a fairly deep S wave in the left-side precordial leads (V_5 and V_6) (Fig. 8–3).

In fact, the R wave in lead V_1 actually becomes taller than the S wave is deep. If we divide the amplitude of the R wave in lead V_1 by the amplitude of the S wave in lead V_1, we normally get a number of less than 1.0. This is called the *R to S ratio* (Fig. 8–4). In RVH, however, the R to S ratio becomes greater than 1.0 because of the exceptionally tall R wave. In other words, the usual pattern of the R wave becoming progressively taller across the precordium from right to left is reversed.

You will recall that in right bundle branch block, we see a similar pattern of a tall R wave in lead V_1 and a deep S wave in lead V_6 (see Fig. 7–3). In order to avoid confusing RVH with right bundle branch block, we must therefore insist that the QRS be of normal duration when diagnosing RVH. The QRS

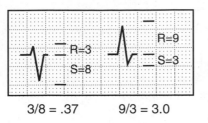

3/8 = .37   9/3 = 3.0

R/S RATIO

Figure 8–4
Calculation of the R to S ratio in any lead.

duration can be in the upper limits of normal, as in LVH, but it cannot be 0.10 second or greater. Nevertheless, a pattern of incomplete right bundle branch block can sometimes be seen with RVH.

The fully developed strain pattern of RVH, like that of LVH, consists of upwardly convex ST depression blending into an inverted T wave, but now it is seen in the right precordial leads (V_1 and V_2), which, of course, look at the right ventricle (Fig. 8–5). The strain pattern may also frequently be seen in those limb leads toward which the main vector of ventricular depolarization is headed (electrical axis). In RVH, this is frequently lead aVF or III because of right axis deviation.

Summary of Criteria for RVH

Remember, again, that the ECG criteria for chamber enlargement have both low sensitivity and low specificity. In summary, these are the things to look for when trying to diagnose right ventricular hypertrophy:

1. R to S ratio of >1.0 in lead V_1 or V_2
2. Right axis deviation
3. Normal QRS duration
4. Strain pattern in lead V_1 or V_2 and in limb leads with the tallest R wave

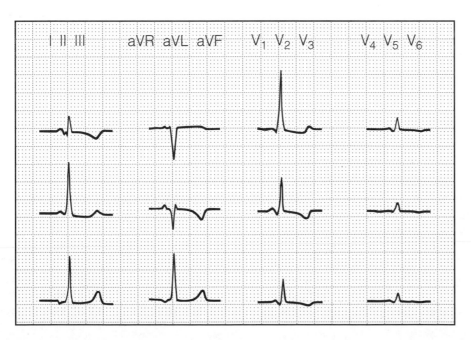

Figure 8–5
Fully developed RVH with a strain pattern in the leads that look at the right ventricle, namely the right-sided precordial leads. This tracing is from a 12-year-old female with congenital heart disease and a single right ventricle.

Practice Tracings

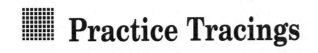

Answers to the practice tracings (Figs. 8–6 and 8–7) on the following pages may be found in the Appendix.

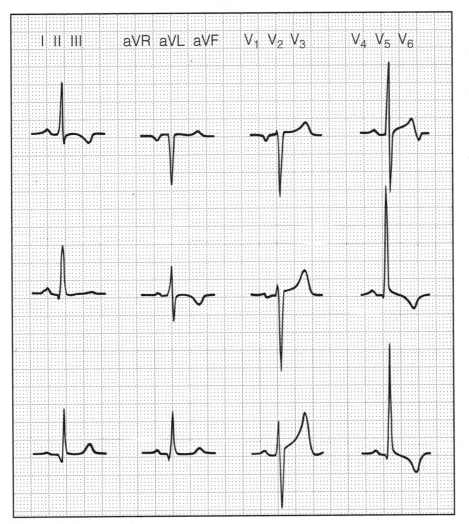

Figure 8–6

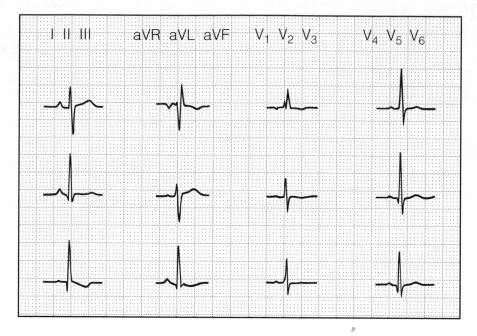

Figure 8–7

Myocardial Infarction

In this chapter, I will discuss what is, for ACLS providers, perhaps the most important and certainly the most clinically interesting subject in 12-lead electrocardiography: acute myocardial infarction.

Anatomy of the Coronary Arteries

The coronary arterial circulation begins with the take-off of the right and left coronary arteries from the aorta. The *left main coronary artery* is very short and rapidly splits into the *left anterior descending artery* and the *circumflex artery*.

The right coronary artery serves primarily the *inferior wall* of the heart; the left anterior descending artery serves the *anterior wall* of the heart; and the circumflex artery serves the *left lateral wall* of the heart. Figure 9–1 illustrates these relationships.

Pathophysiology of Acute Myocardial Infarction

Acute myocardial infarction (AMI) occurs anytime a coronary artery becomes essentially completely obstructed and the segment of myocardium served by that artery loses perfusion and begins to die.

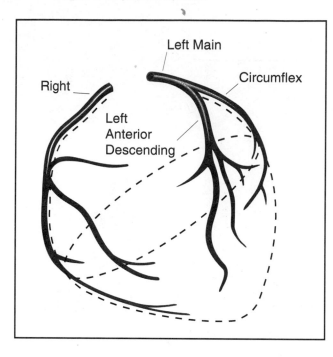

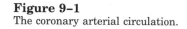

Figure 9–1
The coronary arterial circulation.

Complete obstruction usually occurs in the setting of *fixed obstructive coronary lesions* that are the result of coronary atherosclerosis. However, the process of accumulating *atherosclerotic plaque* in the coronary arteries is slow and gradual. The acute nature of AMI is usually the result of a *clot* forming in the immediate vicinity of an incomplete fixed obstructive lesion. The cause of clot formation may be *rupture* of an atherosclerotic plaque with subsequent platelet aggregation and then clot formation.

Less than complete obstruction of the coronary arteries can produce *ischemia* (diminished perfusion) without actual death of tissue and is the cause of the syndrome labeled *angina*.

Electrocardiographic Hallmarks of Acute Myocardial Infarction

Figure 9–2 illustrates the three ECG hallmarks of *transmural* (through the full thickness of a myocardial wall) AMI:

1. ST segment elevation
2. T wave inversion
3. Q wave formation

These three changes in the ECG typically evolve over a period of minutes to hours, with ST elevation usually appearing first, followed variably by T wave inversion and Q wave formation. Subsequently, the changes may show slow resolution, usually over a period ranging from days to months. Q waves, however, may persist indefinitely, producing ECG evidence of a *scar*.

This sequence of changes is called *electrocardiographic evolution* of an infarction (Fig. 9–3). It is important to recognize that the ECG diagnosis of AMI is much more accurate when made on the basis of evolution over a series of tracings than when made on the basis of a single ECG. Keep in mind also

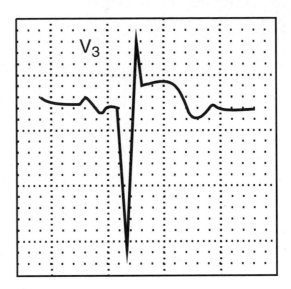

Figure 9–2
The three electrocardiographic hallmarks of acute myocardial infarction (AMI), including ST elevation, T wave inversion, and Q wave formation.

that the ECG may not reveal clear patterns of infarction in the earliest stages of evolution.

You may have deduced from the above discussion that it is extremely important to correlate clinical signs and symptoms with the ECG before making the diagnosis of AMI. More on that later.

Figure 9–3
Evolution of an inferior wall myocardial infarction (MI) as seen in lead III of a 55-year-old white male. Note that the admission tracing shows only ST elevation. A Q wave is beginning to form by 1 hour, and ST elevation is on the way down. By 24 hours, Q wave formation is complete and the T wave is fully inverted. By 1 year, a pathologic Q wave is the only remaining evidence of infarction.

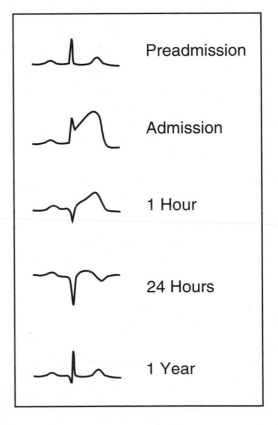

Localization of Infarction

It is often possible to determine in a general way which wall of the heart is involved in an infarction by determining in which leads we see the three hallmarks of AMI.

You will recall from Chapter 3 and from your knowledge of the hexaxial reference system (Fig. 9–4) that leads II, III, and aVF are called the inferior leads because they look up at the heart from below. When the typical evolution of the three hallmarks of AMI is seen in leads II, III, and aVF, we label it an *inferior wall myocardial infarction* (MI).

If the ST elevation, T wave inversion, and Q wave formation are seen in leads I and aVL, we call it a *lateral wall infarction* because leads I and aVL look at the lateral wall of the heart.

Finally, if we see evolutionary changes across leads V_2, V_3, and V_4, we label it *anterior wall infarction* because the precordial leads look at the anterior wall of the heart.

Either inferior or anterior wall infarctions can also sometimes show changes in the far lateral precordial leads (V_5 and V_6) as well as in leads I and aVL. The descriptive terms *inferolateral* and *anterolateral* are then used to locate the infarction.

Electrocardiographers usually require that the changes of infarction be seen in two or more *contiguous leads* (adjacent leads) on the hexaxial reference system or among the precordial leads before a diagnosis of infarction is made. For example, to diagnose an inferior wall infarction, one would have to see changes in at least leads II and aVF, or in leads aVF and III, because each of these pairs of leads are contiguous.

ST Elevation

ST elevation in AMI occurs in the presence of myocardium that is in the process of dying, and it is often called a *current of injury*. Note in Figure 9–2 that the ST elevation of AMI is typically, but not always, *upwardly convex*, meaning that it bows upward. This produces an appearance that some have likened to that of a fireman's cap. ST elevation may also be upwardly concave, however.

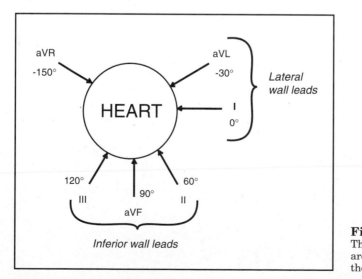

Figure 9–4
The hexaxial reference system showing those leads that are considered to reflect the inferior and lateral walls of the heart.

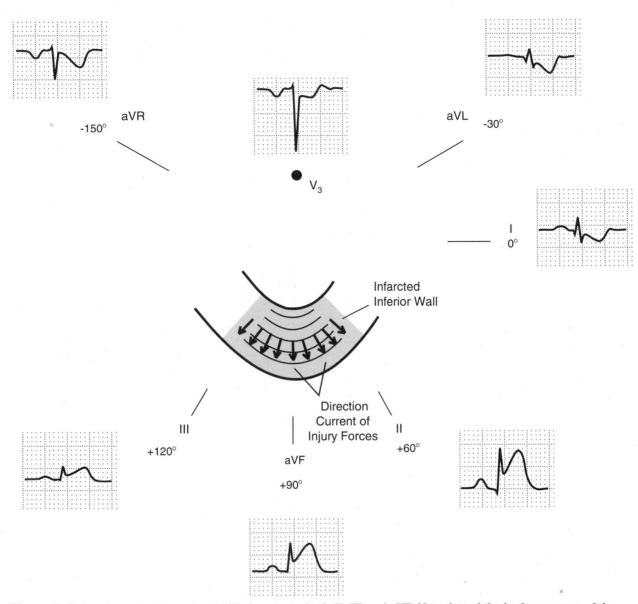

Figure 9–5. Inferior wall AMI producing ST elevation in leads II, III, and aVF. Note that while the force vectors of the current of injury are coming toward II, III, and aVF, they are going away from the reciprocal leads of I and aVL and the precordial leads represented in the diagram by V₃. The deviation of the ECG needle is therefore negative in the reciprocal leads, producing what is called reciprocal ST depression.

Because ST elevation is an upward deflection of the ECG needle, it is clear that the current of injury in the infarcted wall of myocardium is producing force vectors similar to those of a T wave that are coming toward the lead in which we view the ST elevation.

In Figure 9–5 we see the force vectors of a current of injury in the inferior wall coming toward leads II, III, and aVF and producing ST elevation in those leads. By the same token, the force vectors are going away from the leads in the *reciprocal* or opposite leads I and aVL and the precordial leads V₂ through V₄, represented in the diagram by V₃. This produces what is called *reciprocal depression* in the wall of the heart opposite the location of the infarction.

Thus, inferior wall MIs produce reciprocal depression in the anterior and high lateral walls (leads V₂ through V₄ and I and aVL). Anterior MIs produce reciprocal depression in the inferior wall (leads II, III, and aVF) as shown in Figure 9–6.

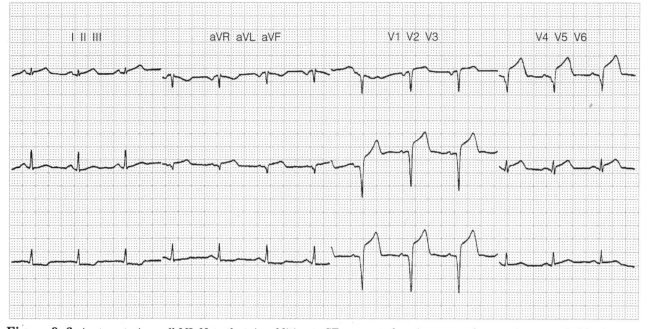

Figure 9–6. Acute anterior wall MI. Note that, in addition to ST segment elevation across the anterior precordial leads, there is reciprocal depression seen in leads III and aVF. Note also that, in this particular patient, the ST elevation is slightly upwardly concave.

Classic reciprocal depression does not always appear with the ST elevation of AMI, however. Reciprocal depression is fleeting, and depending on the timing of the tracing, a substantial number of AMIs may not show it. When present, however, reciprocal depression greatly enhances the confidence with which one can label an infarction as acute.

When ST elevation alone is seen without other confirming evidence of AMI, most electrocardiographers require that at least 1 mm of elevation be seen in two or more contiguous limb leads for diagnosis of inferior infarctions and at least 2 mm in two or more contiguous precordial leads for diagnosis of anterior wall infarctions.

ST elevation itself is not confined exclusively to AMI. Other conditions can cause ST elevation, including pericarditis and ventricular aneurysm. ST elevation can even be seen as a normal variant in healthy people. There are ways, however, to differentiate these other causes of ST elevation from AMI. These methods will be discussed later in this chapter under the heading Differential Diagnosis of ST Elevation.

T Wave Inversion

As the ST elevation seen in AMI begins to come down, the T wave also begins to come down from its upright position and eventually inverts. In the intermediate position, it is frequently biphasic. Figure 9–7 shows an anterolateral wall infarction, substantially along in evolution, with slight remaining ST elevation and prominent T wave inversion in leads V_2 through V_5 and I and aVL.

Q Wave Formation

When a segment of myocardium undergoes infarction, it ceases to depolarize normally and becomes essentially *electrically inert.* As a result, there are no forces of ventricular depolarization spreading from endocardium to epicar-

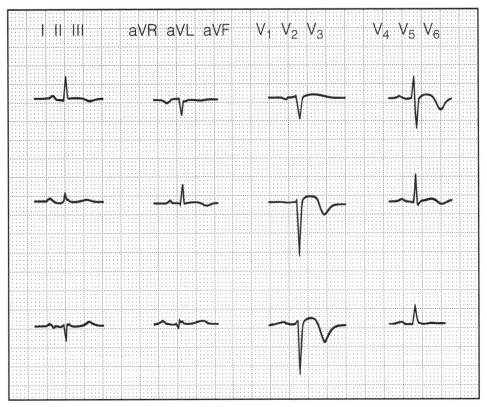

Figure 9–7. Evolving anterior wall MI showing loss of R wave progression in leads V_2 through V_4. Slight ST elevation remains, and there is prominent T wave inversion in leads V_2 through V_5 and I and aVL.

dium and coming directly toward whichever leads are viewing the infarcted wall. Instead, the leads viewing the infarction are looking through the "window" of inactive infarcted myocardium at the forces of the opposite wall of the ventricle. These vectors in the opposite wall are also spreading from endocardium to epicardium and are therefore going away from the leads looking at the infarction. This concept of an electrical window through the infarction looking on the "back wall" of the heart, as illustrated in Figure 9–8, is a simplified but useful concept for explaining Q wave formation in the leads looking at the infarction.

In an anterior wall infarction, for example, as the anterior wall begins to die, the forces of anterior wall depolarization gradually decline until they cease. As a result, the R wave normally seen in the anterior precordial leads gradually becomes smaller and smaller until the initial deflection finally becomes a Q. This is called *loss of R wave progression* across the precordium. Figure 9–7 shows substantial loss of the normal R wave in leads V_2 through V_4, but actual Q wave formation has not yet occurred. Figure 9–6 shows full Q wave formation in leads V_1 through V_5.

You will recall from our previous discussion of the normal ECG that as a result of septal depolarization, a small Q wave is often normally seen in the inferior leads II, III, and aVF. With acute inferior wall infarction, the Q becomes deeper and wider until it reaches criteria for becoming what electrocardiographers call a *pathologic Q wave*. Most electrocardiographers define a pathologic Q wave as being at least 0.04 second wide with a depth greater than 25% of the height of the R wave. Thus, the presence of a Q wave alone in the inferior leads is not enough to diagnose an inferior wall infarction, unless the Q wave is pathologic. Figure 9–9 shows an acute inferior wall MI with pathologic Q wave formation along with ST elevation in leads II, III, and aVF.

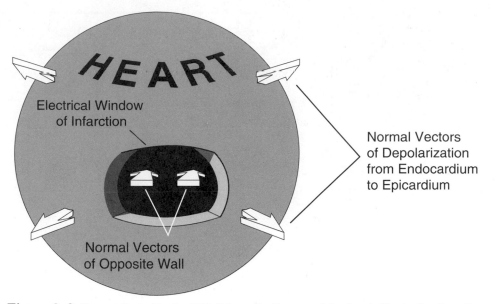

Figure 9–8. Q wave formation in AMI. Schematic diagram of the heart, illustrating how the "window" of electrically inert infarcted tissue in AMI permits the electrode viewing the infarction to look through the window at the opposite wall of the heart. Normal force vectors in the opposite wall are going away from the electrode, traveling from endocardium to epicardium, producing a negative deflection, which we call a Q wave.

Q Waves as Scars

It was mentioned earlier in the chapter that the ST elevation and T wave inversion seen in AMI frequently resolve over time but the Q wave may persist indefinitely as evidence of a past infarction. Pathologic Q waves in the absence of AMI are therefore sometimes referred to in ECG reports as *scars* or *remote infarctions*. Figures 9–10 and 9–11 show remote inferior and anterior infarctions, respectively, in which the ST elevation and T wave inversion have resolved but Q waves persist as evidence of the old infarction. Close inspection of the acute inferior MI shown in Figure 9–9 also reveals a pathologic Q wave in leads V_1 and V_2, indicating an old anterior wall infarction.

Non–Q Wave Infarctions

Sometimes in AMI, if the infarction is small or if it does not involve the full thickness of the myocardial wall, an actual Q wave never develops. This is called *non–Q wave*, or *subendocardial, infarction.*

In anterior wall non–Q wave infarctions, we may see loss of R wave progression, even though the Q wave never forms. With inferior wall non–Q wave infarctions, either a Q wave never forms or the normal Q wave, if present, simply never becomes deep enough or wide enough to meet criteria for a pathologic Q wave.

Non–Q wave infarctions, therefore, must be diagnosed electrocardiographically solely on the basis of evolution in the ST segment and T wave. Only approximately one third of patients with non–Q wave infarctions ever develop ST elevation. The remaining two thirds develop ST depression alone and subsequent T wave inversion. Figure 9–12 shows a non–Q wave infarction of the anterior wall with deep T wave inversion across the precordium but no loss of R wave.

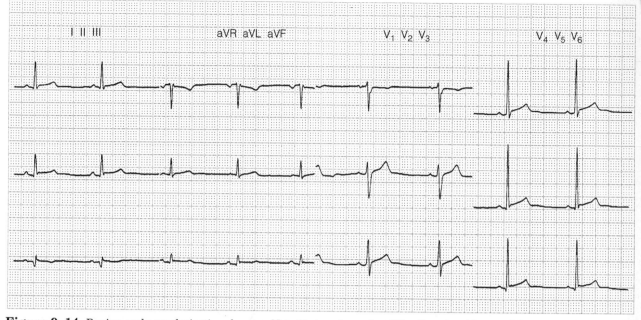
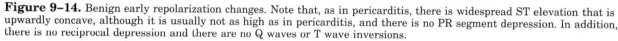

Figure 9–14. Benign early repolarization changes. Note that, as in pericarditis, there is widespread ST elevation that is upwardly concave, although it is usually not as high as in pericarditis, and there is no PR segment depression. In addition, there is no reciprocal depression and there are no Q waves or T wave inversions.

Other Pitfalls in Diagnosing Acute Myocardial Infarction

Earlier in this chapter it was mentioned that observing the evolution of AMI on serial ECG tracings leads to more accurate diagnosis of AMI than does reading of a single tracing. One of the reasons for this is that occasionally ST segment elevation may persist for many months after AMI. This is particularly true of large anterior infarctions. Indeed, the ECG diagnosis of a *ventricular aneurysm* is based upon ST elevation persisting indefinitely after AMI (Fig. 9–15). It is therefore easy to mistakenly conclude on the basis of a single random ECG that a patient with a ventricular aneurysm is in the process of having an AMI, when in actuality the infarction may be months or years old.

A clue to the age of the infarction shown in Figure 9–15 is that there is no reciprocal depression. The absence of reciprocal depression is characteristic of old infarctions that demonstrate persistent ST elevation. When there is a question of whether an ECG infarction pattern is new or old, the presence of reciprocal depression lends strong support to the conclusion that the infarction is acute. Conversely, the absence of reciprocal depression should raise the question in the reader's mind of whether observed ST elevation may actually represent ventricular aneurysm as the result of a remote infarction. The best way to deal with this question of age is always to compare the current tracing with a previous one on file and to lay heavy emphasis on correlation of the current ECG with the clinical picture.

Another potential pitfall in the diagnosis of AMI lies in patients with left bundle branch block (LBBB). As shown in Figure 9–16, LBBB produces Q waves in the anterior precordial leads along with upward slurring of the ST segment. This combination can simulate acute anterior wall infarction. However, the converse is also true. Some patients with extensive anterior wall infarctions develop LBBB because of extensive necrosis of the septum. Indeed, diagnosing AMI in patients with LBBB is so fraught with peril that the safest course is never to try to make an ECG diagnosis of AMI in patients with LBBB.

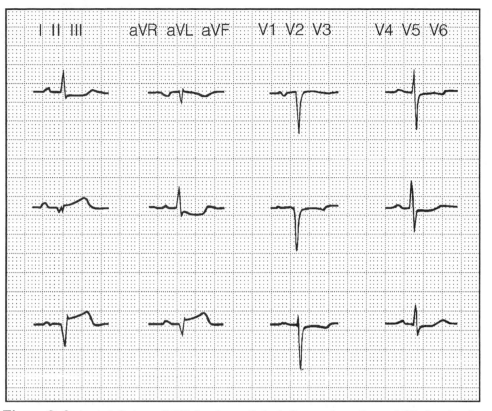

Figure 9–9. Acute inferior wall MI showing pathologic Q wave formation and ST elevation in leads II, III, and aVF. A pathologic Q wave can also be seen in leads V_1 and V_2, denoting an old anterior wall infarction.

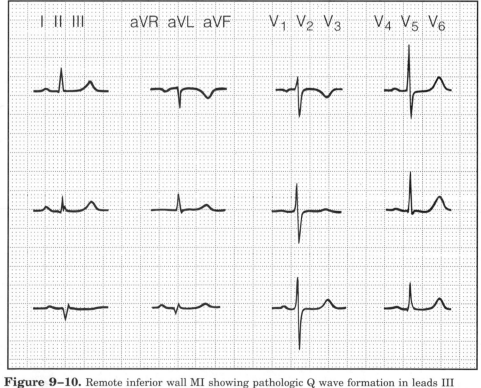

Figure 9–10. Remote inferior wall MI showing pathologic Q wave formation in leads III and aVF.

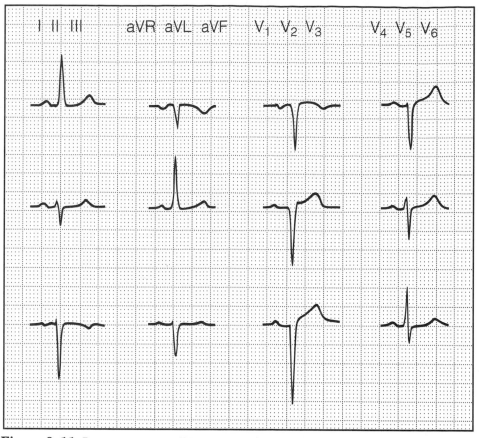

Figure 9–11. Remote anterior wall MI showing pathologic Q wave formation in leads V₁ through V₃. Although there is still slight ST elevation that has persisted, as is sometimes the case with large infarctions, note that there is no reciprocal depression in the inferior leads and that T waves in the anterior wall are upright.

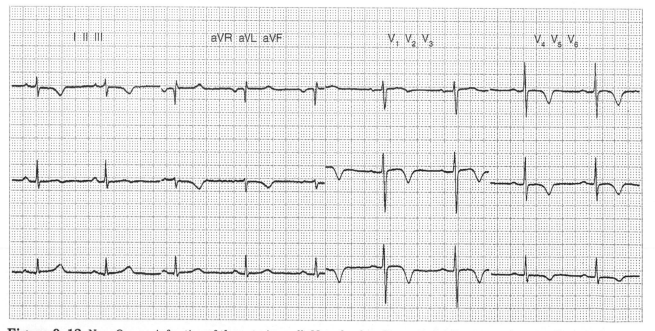

Figure 9–12. Non–Q wave infarction of the anterior wall. Note the deep T wave inversion across the precordium and the absence of Q waves.

Differential Diagnosis of ST Elevation

Acute myocardial infarction is not the only condition that can cause ST segment elevation. Several other conditions, including *pericarditis* and *benign early repolarization changes* (a normal variant of ST elevation seen commonly in healthy young adults), routinely produce ST elevation. It is important, therefore, to distinguish AMI from other causes of ST elevation.

Several distinguishing criteria can be helpful. First, as described earlier in this chapter, the ST elevation of AMI is often accompanied by reciprocal depression in the wall opposite the infarction. Pericarditis and benign early repolarization changes, however, show no reciprocal depression but do typically show ST elevation in all walls. In other words, the ST elevation is not localized to one wall but is widespread and is reflected in more than one electrocardiographic region of the heart.

Figure 9–13 shows the tracing of a young adult male with acute pericarditis. Note that the ST elevation is widespread throughout the inferior, anterior, and lateral walls, and there is no reciprocal depression. Another very helpful clue that this tracing represents pericarditis rather than AMI is the presence of *PR segment depression*. Note that the PR segment shows slightly downsloping depression in all leads. This finding is characteristic of pericarditis.

Figure 9–14 is the tracing of a healthy, asymptomatic 34-year-old male who has no clinical evidence of pericardial or myocardial disease. This tracing is typical of benign early repolarization changes and, as in pericarditis, shows widespread ST elevation without reciprocal depression. Unlike findings with pericarditis, however, there is no PR segment depression.

A second helpful distinguishing criterion between AMI and these other two causes of ST elevation is that the ST segment elevation of AMI is typically upwardly convex or only very slightly concave. Note in Figures 9–13 and 9–14, however, that the ST elevation of pericarditis and benign early repolarization changes are typically *deeply concave*.

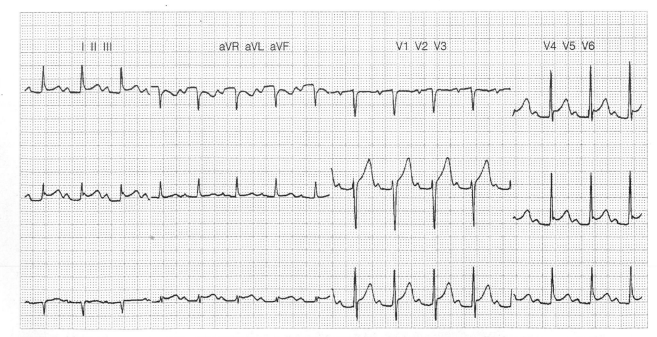

Figure 9–13. Acute pericarditis. Note that there is widespread ST elevation that is upwardly deeply concave in the anterior, inferior, and lateral walls. In addition, there is no reciprocal depression and there are no Q waves. PR segment depression is also present.

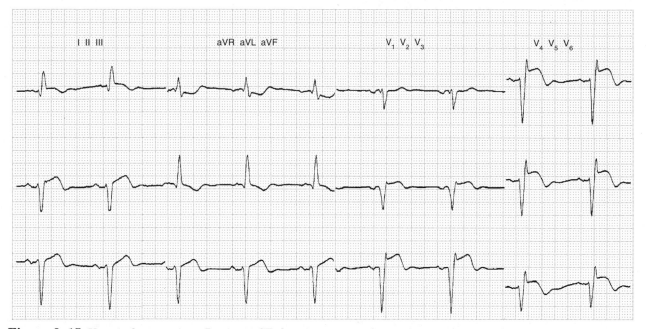

Figure 9–15. Ventricular aneurysm. Persistent ST elevation 4 years after acute anterior wall infarction in a 75-year-old male with aneurysm of the left ventricle proven by echocardiogram. Note the absence of reciprocal depression as one of the clues that this infarction may be old. An incidental intraventricular conduction delay is also present.

In this situation, the clinical presentation becomes all-important, as discussed in Chapter 11.

A final pitfall worthy of consideration is the presence of left anterior hemiblock (LAH) as discussed at length in Chapter 6. Figures 6–6 and 6–7 demonstrate that the extreme left axis deviation of LAH can be mistaken for the Q waves of remote inferior wall infarction if one does not search carefully for the tiny R waves in leads II, III, and aVF that are part of the criteria for LAH.

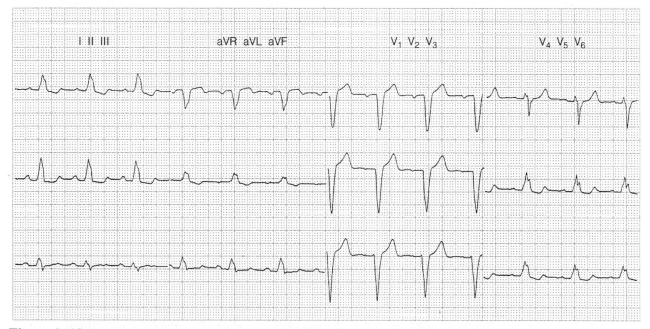

Figure 9–16. LBBB simulating anterior wall infarction. Q waves in V_2 and V_3 together with upward slurring of the ST segments can often be mistaken for acute anterior wall infarction if one does not notice that the QRS duration is 0.12 second or greater and that there is an RSR′ in the lateral precordial leads.

Practice Tracings

The tracings in Figures 9–17 to 9–20 are for practicing your new skills at diagnosing myocardial infarction. The answers may be found in the Appendix.

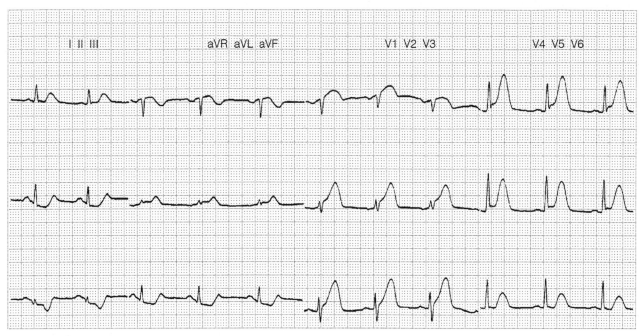

Figure 9–17

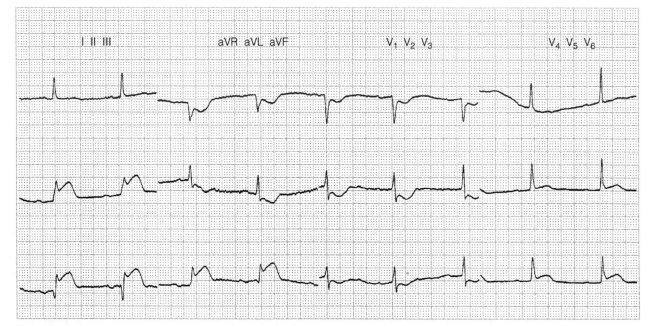

Figure 9–18

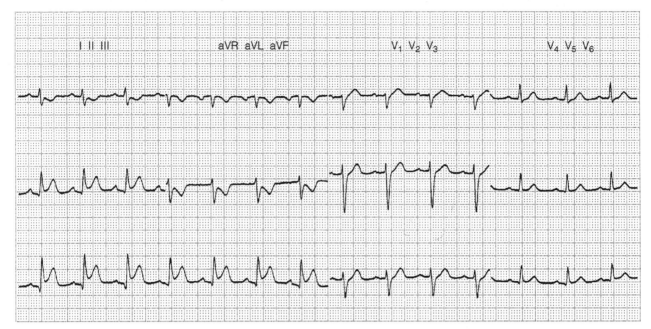

Figure 9-19

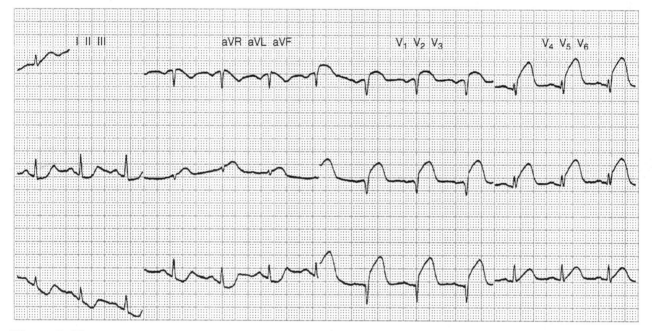

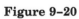

Figure 9-20

Ischemia and Anginal Syndromes

Not all instances of diminished coronary artery perfusion result in myocardial infarction. In this chapter, I will discuss electrocardiographic findings in less-than-complete coronary artery obstruction.

Pathophysiology of Ischemia

When arterial perfusion of tissue is inadequate to meet metabolic needs, we say that the tissue is *ischemic*. Metabolic needs in the case of a muscle are dependent upon the workload of that muscle.

In coronary artery disease, incomplete obstruction of the coronary arteries with atherosclerotic plaque limits myocardial perfusion. Under circumstances of rest, the diminished flow of oxygenated arterial blood may still be sufficient to meet the metabolic needs of the myocardium. However, during periods of exercise, the needs of the myocardium may require a greater volume of blood than can be delivered through the partially obstructed coronary arteries. In short, *myocardial oxygen consumption* may outstrip oxygen supply. The result is ischemia of the myocardium.

Anginal Syndromes

If the patient has chest pain in association with ischemia occurring during exercise, the syndrome is labeled *exertional angina pectoris*. Typically, when the patient rests, the imbalance between oxygen supply and demand resolves and the pain goes away.

Exercise is not the only circumstance under which angina can occur, however. Any circumstance that increases heart rate or blood pressure—for example, anxiety or a large meal—may increase myocardial oxygen consumption and result in angina.

Myocardial ischemia can also occur without producing chest pain. Many patients with coronary artery disease have frequent periods of *silent ischemia* occurring in the absence of chest pain.

Coronary artery spasm is another cause of myocardial ischemia, sometimes occurring even in patients with completely clean coronary arteries. More often, however, spasm occurs in the immediate vicinity of atherosclerotic plaque in patients with severe coronary artery disease. Spasm diminishes perfusion and can produce exactly the same ischemic consequences as atherosclerosis.

Some patients with coronary artery spasm typically develop their pain at night during sleep and demonstrate reversible ST elevation on their ECG during pain rather than the ST depression that is typical of most forms of angina. This syndrome has been labeled *variant angina* or *Prinzmetal's angina*.

Often in clinical practice, we see patients who have prolonged periods of ischemic chest pain at rest but who do not demonstrate evidence of acute myocardial infarction. This syndrome is called *unstable angina*. It typically occurs in patients with a very severe fixed stenosis or narrowing of a coronary artery, often exceeding a 90% obstruction. Sometimes a thrombus at the site of the stenosis intermittently further narrows or occludes the lumen. A high percentage of affected patients will go on to develop acute myocardial infarction.

Electrophysiologic Changes During Ischemia

During periods of ischemia, blood flow diminishes first and most dramatically in the subendocardium. Epicardial blood flow is preserved until the artery supplying the affected muscle becomes almost completely obstructed. As a result, ischemia usually involves only a partial thickness of the ventricular wall.

Significant metabolic changes occur in the ischemic inner wall (subendocardium), while the metabolic state of the outer wall (epicardium) remains nearly normal. This creates a difference in electrical potential between ischemic and normal tissue with the net result that there is a current flow from normal cells in the epicardium toward the ischemic cells in the endocardium (Fig. 10–1). This current flow takes place during mechanical systole, which, as you know from Chapter 1, occupies the time interval of the ST segment. Since the current is flowing away from ECG electrodes on the body surface overlying the affected ventricular wall, it is registered on the ECG as a negative needle deflection, resulting in *ST depression*. As you would surmise, these same electrophysiologic events can also alter T waves.

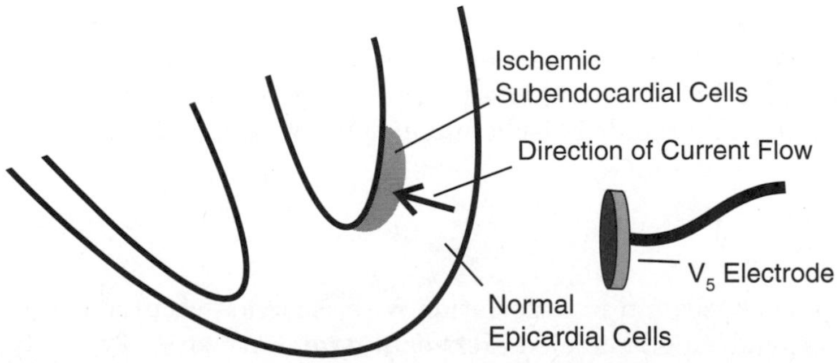

Ischemic Subendocardial Cells

Direction of Current Flow

V_5 Electrode

Normal Epicardial Cells

Figure 10–1
Schematic view of the left ventricle showing the flow of current during systole from healthy cells in the epicardium toward ischemic cells in the subendocardium. Note that the current flow is away from the V_5 electrode, producing a negative deflection of the ECG needle, which results in ST depression.

When ischemia involves the full thickness of the ventricular wall, that is, both endocardium and epicardium, we say that it is *transmural*. As noted above, this requires almost total cessation of blood flow through a coronary artery. *Transmural ischemia* produces ST elevation, with which you are already familiar from your study of acute myocardial infarction (Chapter 9).

Characteristics of Ischemic ST Depression

The ST segment depression seen with nontransmural ischemia typically is either horizontal (flat) or downsloping, and the ST segment is usually quite straight, as shown in Figure 10–2. Note also that the ST segment in ischemia typically intersects with the T wave at a fairly abrupt angle. Both the straight ST segment and the abrupt transition into the T wave are in contrast to other causes of ST depression. Left ventricular hypertrophy, for example, has downsloping ST depression, but it is typically upwardly convex, and there is a gentle transition into the T wave (Fig. 10–3).

Upsloping ST depression, on the other hand, much less often represents ischemia and, in fact, is quite normal during periods of exercise or other causes of tachycardia. This normal exertional ST depression is often referred to as *J-point depression* (Fig. 10–4).

ST depression is measured from the isoelectric line, usually established by the PR segment. As a general rule, the deeper the ST depression, the more severe the ischemia. In addition, the deeper the ST depression, the greater the specificity for ischemia. ST depression of less than 1 mm is an unreliable indicator of ischemia. Figure 10–5 shows the full 12-lead ECG of a patient with severe ischemia during an anginal attack.

Intermittent ST Depression

As you learned earlier in this chapter, ischemia is usually a changing, dynamic state that comes and goes, depending upon the current balance or imbalance between oxygen supply and demand in the tissues. By the same token, ST depression is also often transient. It comes and goes with the ischemic

Figure 10–2
Ischemia. Horizontal ST segment depression associated with ischemia. Note that the ST segment is quite straight and intersects with the T wave at a fairly sharp angle.

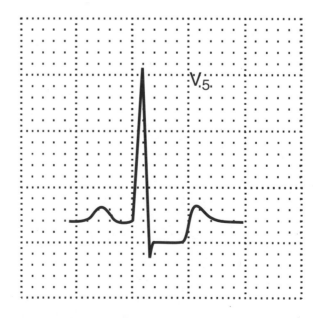

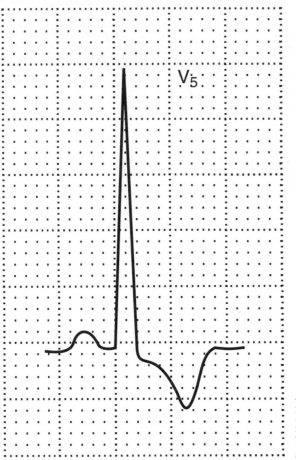

Figure 10–3
Left ventricular hypertrophy (LVH). Note that the ST depression
in LVH is downsloping, as it can be in ischemia,
but that the ST segment is convex as opposed to straight and
gently blends into the T wave.

state. Many patients with severe coronary artery disease display perfectly
normal ECGs at rest and demonstrate ST depression only when ischemia is
precipitated by exercise or occurs during an anginal episode. This fact gave
rise to *exercise stress testing* as a means of detecting occlusive coronary artery
disease in patients with normal resting ECGs. During stress testing, a 12-lead
ECG is continuously monitored while the patient walks on a treadmill or
peddles a stationary bicycle. Any ischemia provoked by exercise is then detected

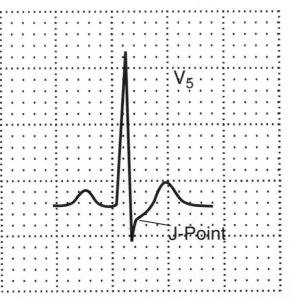

Figure 10–4
J-point depression. Upsloping ST depression from the J-point that
is a physiologic response to exercise or tachycardia.

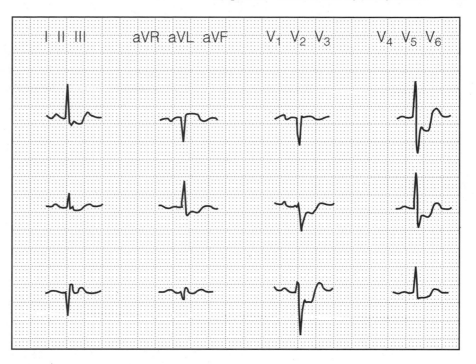

Figure 10–5
Ischemia. ECG of a 76-year-old white male recorded during an episode of angina. Note up to 3 mm of horizontal or downsloping ST depression in the anterolateral wall. In addition, pathologic Q waves are present in leads III and aVF, reflecting a previous inferior wall infarction.

by observing for horizontal or downsloping ST depression of greater than 1 mm. Care must be taken not to falsely interpret physiologic J-point depression as representing ischemia.

Figure 10–6A shows the tracing of a 51-year-old white male with a normal resting ECG, diagnostic ST depression occurring at 10.5 minutes into exercise, and resolution of ST changes by 4 minutes into the postexercise period.

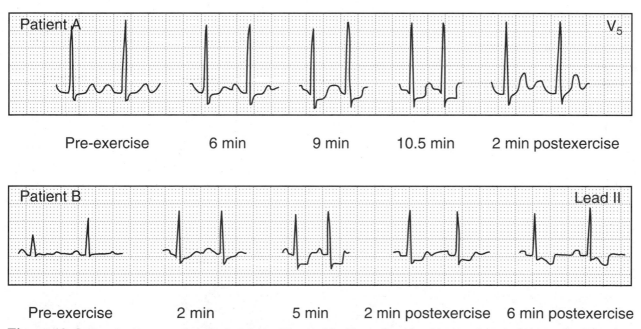

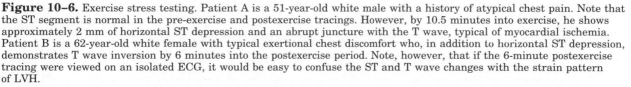

Figure 10–6. Exercise stress testing. Patient A is a 51-year-old white male with a history of atypical chest pain. Note that the ST segment is normal in the pre-exercise and postexercise tracings. However, by 10.5 minutes into exercise, he shows approximately 2 mm of horizontal ST depression and an abrupt juncture with the T wave, typical of myocardial ischemia. Patient B is a 62-year-old white female with typical exertional chest discomfort who, in addition to horizontal ST depression, demonstrates T wave inversion by 6 minutes into the postexercise period. Note, however, that if the 6-minute postexercise tracing were viewed on an isolated ECG, it would be easy to confuse the ST and T wave changes with the strain pattern of LVH.

Chronic ST Depression

Some patients with coronary artery disease have persistent imbalances between oxygen supply and demand that are reflected as *chronic ST depression* on the ECG. Thus, these patients display ST depression even on the resting ECG in the absence of pain (Fig. 10–7).

T Wave Inversion

As briefly mentioned earlier in this chapter, the flow of current from normal myocardial cells in the epicardium toward ischemic cells in the subendocardium during systole can also change repolarization sequences, resulting in T wave abnormalities. Thus, *T wave inversion,* although seen less frequently than ST depression, is another potential indicator of ischemia. T wave inversion may accompany ST depression, or it may be seen alone as a manifestation of ischemia. Figure 10-6B shows T wave inversion occurring postexercise in a 62-year-old white female with typical exertional chest discomfort and a positive stress exercise test for ischemia. Note, however, that the upwardly convex nature of the ST depression gently sloping into an inverted T wave could easily be confused with left ventricular hypertrophy if viewed on an isolated ECG. Thus, T wave inversion is a less reliable indicator of ischemia than is horizontal ST depression.

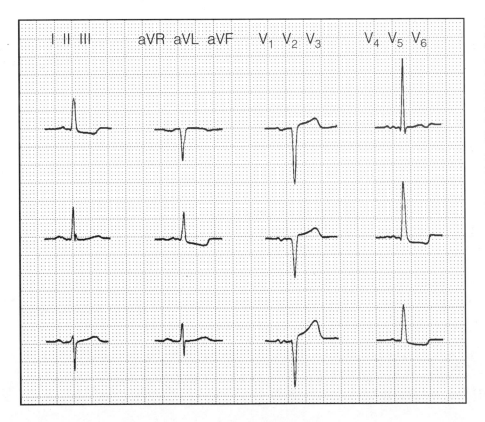

Figure 10–7
Chronic ST depression. This 76-year-old male patient demonstrates chronic ST depression that persists from tracing to tracing in the high lateral wall (leads I, aVL, V_5, and V_6). Note that the downsloping ST depression forms an abrupt angle with the T wave and that the T wave itself is altered by the ischemia. This patient also demonstrates evidence of a previous anterior MI in the form of pathologic Q waves in leads V_1 through V_3.

Differential Diagnosis of ST Abnormalities

It should be clear by now that there are many conditions that can affect ST segments and T waves, including bundle branch block, acute myocardial infarction, chamber enlargement, and ischemia. You will learn of even more in Chapter 12 (Miscellaneous Conditions). A frequent reader of ECGs will also see many tracings with mild ST abnormalities that can only be called *nonspecific ST and T wave changes* because they are not clearly characteristic of any of the conditions referred to above (Fig. 10–8).

A few hints can be helpful in sorting out these sometimes difficult differentiations. With regard to ischemia, perhaps the most helpful clue when evaluating ST and T wave abnormalities is whether or not they change from tracing to tracing. Conditions like bundle branch block and left ventricular hypertrophy are persistent and do not change much over a period of time. Ischemic ST depression, however, frequently changes from tracing to tracing. Thus, as usual, it is a good idea, whenever possible, to compare the current tracing with an old tracing on file to see if noted changes are acute or chronic.

The straightness of the ST segment and the acuteness of the angle with the T wave are highly significant criteria when evaluating ST depression, and their presence makes the changes more likely to be ischemic in origin.

Finally, clinical correlation, as always, is also helpful. For example, ST depression appearing with chest pain and resolving when the chest pain resolves makes the diagnosis of ischemia a virtual certainty. The clinical and ECG correlates of ischemic heart disease are the subject of our next chapter.

Figure 10–8
Nonspecific ST segment changes. Note that the sagging ST segments and minimal T wave inversion in the inferior and lateral walls are not clearly characteristic of any specific category of ST segment abnormality or T wave abnormality, and thus the designation "nonspecific."

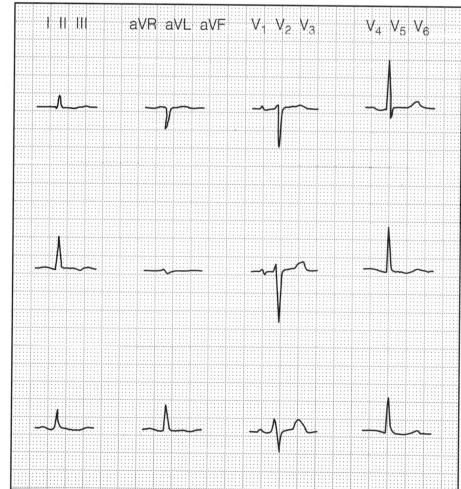

Practice Tracings

Several practice tracings (Figs. 10–9 to 10–12) are included on this and the next page for honing your skills in diagnosing myocardial ischemia. The answers may be found in the Appendix.

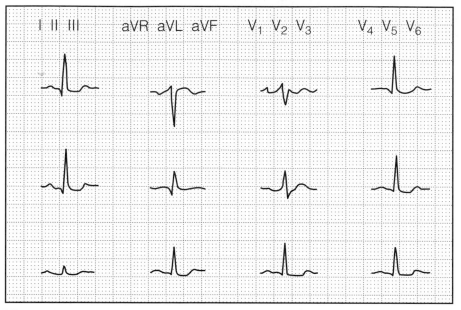

Figure 10–9

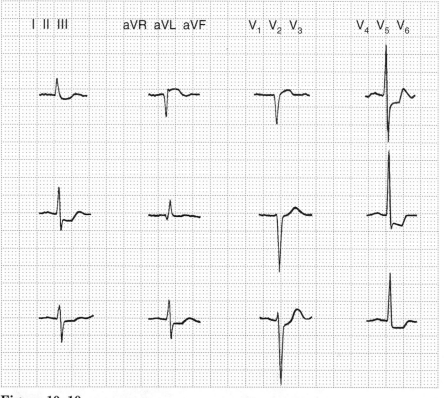

Figure 10–10

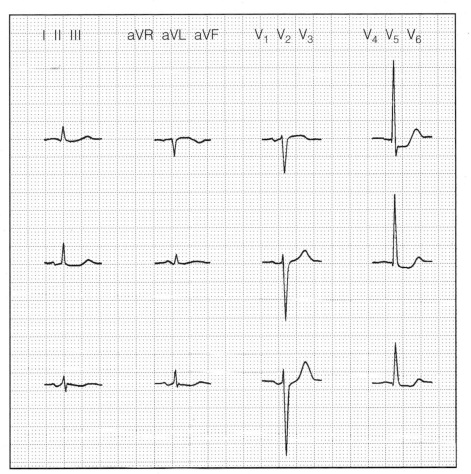

Figure 10–11

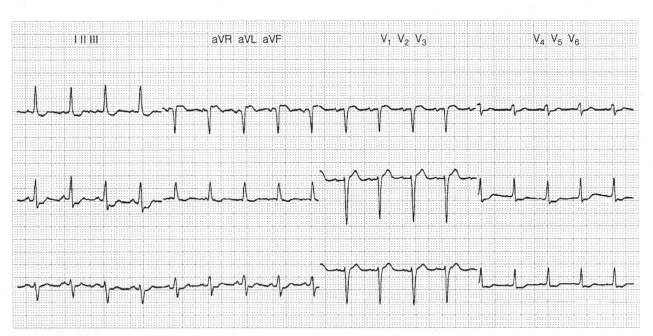

Figure 10–12

The ECG and the Clinical Evaluation of Chest Pain

Interpretation of the 12-lead electrocardiogram is always more accurate when the ECG is correlated with the patient's clinical presentation. In this chapter, I will discuss the various clinical syndromes of ischemic heart disease, the approach to the patient with chest pain, and the use of the ECG in chest pain evaluation.

The Electrocardiogram as a Tool

Because there are often several conditions that can produce similar changes in the ECG, it is usually a mistake to rely on the ECG alone in making a diagnosis. Rather, the ECG should be considered as just one of many pieces of evidence that must be weighed in reaching an accurate clinical diagnosis. It is always important to interpret the ECG in light of the patient's clinical presentation.

For example, in Figure 9–14, you saw that patients with ventricular aneurysms frequently have persistent ST elevation that sometimes cannot easily be distinguished from that caused by an acute infarction. It would be very easy to mistakenly conclude that such a patient was having an acute infarction unless we noted that the patient was free of pain and had no symptoms compatible with acute myocardial infarction.

Correlation of the ECG with the clinical presentation is never more important than when approaching the patient with potential ischemic heart disease. In this chapter, I will discuss in detail the clinical presentation of the various syndromes associated with ischemic heart disease and the clinical approach to this group of patients.

The Role of History Taking

The clinical presentation of pain resulting from ischemic heart disease remains one of the most diverse in medicine. Nevertheless, studies have demonstrated that a history taken by an experienced clinician is a more accurate predictor of ischemic heart disease than is any single available test, with the exception of coronary arteriography. For this reason, an accurate history taken by a well-trained ACLS provider is paramount to the evaluation of the patient presenting with chest pain. In most instances, it is the history that will trigger the provider's decision to move the patient along a path of evaluation for ischemic heart disease.

Syndromes of Ischemic Heart Disease

The continuum of ischemic heart disease stretches from silent ischemia through the various patterns of angina, acute myocardial infarction, and scars of a previous myocardial infarction to the complications of acute myocardial infarction, such as ventricular aneurysm or pericarditis. Although all of these syndromes represent a continuum of the same disease process, they may present with quite different ECG patterns and have distinctly different treatment and outcomes.

When patients present with chest pain, the ECG can help us to determine where they fit on the continuum. Similarly, the nature of the symptoms and the physical examination can provide clues as to where the patients fit on the continuum and can lead us to search for subtle ECG changes that we might otherwise overlook without a high index of suspicion.

Stable Angina

Stable exertional angina, occurring predictably with a given level of exercise, is the most common initial presentation of ischemic heart disease. Discomfort appears with a fairly predictable and reproducible level of exercise, such as walking briskly for half a block, and just as predictably fades within several minutes with rest or nitroglycerin. The discomfort is variously described as a pressure, tightness, weight, band around the chest, indigestion, or gas. It may be felt in the epigastrium, retrosternally, in the arms, shoulders, neck, or jaws.

Occasionally, shortness of breath with exertion (in the absence of chronic lung disease) may be the only manifestation of angina. Nausea, vomiting, and diaphoresis are usually absent with angina.

Pathologically, stable angina is characterized by fixed obstructive coronary disease, usually requiring greater than a 50% stenosis. The prognosis for stable angina is quite good, and usually no emergency treatment other than sublingual nitroglycerin is required.

The ECG may or may not show evidence of ischemia, depending upon the timing of the tracing. As you learned in Chapter 10, many patients with angina have prefectly normal ECG tracings in the absence of pain. It is important to remember that a normal tracing in a patient whose pain has resolved does not rule out the diagnosis of angina. Every attempt should be made to perform the ECG while the patient has pain.

Unstable Angina/Intermediate Syndrome

Unstable angina is characterized by any change from a previous stable pattern of angina or by new onset of angina. Frequent manifestations include discomfort coming with less and less exertion, and discomfort coming at rest, lasting longer, or requiring more nitroglycerin for relief.

Duration of discomfort is frequently longer than with stable angina and may last as long as an hour or more without the patient's developing evidence of acute myocardial infarction. Nausea, vomiting, and diaphoresis are still typically absent, although, as with stable angina, shortness of breath may occasionally be present.

An interesting and not uncommon pattern is that of angina that occurs with the patient at rest after lying down and is relieved by the patient's sitting up or walking around the room. This *recumbent* or *nocturnal angina* is thought to be due to an increase in cardiac work that occurs in the recumbent position because of increased venous return. Although recumbent angina usually represents a relatively severe degree of stenosis, there are patients for whom it represents a stable pattern, and it does not necessarily represent unstable angina.

Pathologically, unstable angina, sometimes called the *intermediate syndrome* when associated with prolonged pain, is typically characterized by severe fixed obstructive disease with stenosis often in excess of 90%. Evidence is also accumulating that incomplete coronary thrombosis may play a role in unstable angina.

Patients with unstable angina and the intermediate syndrome are at much higher risk of progressing to myocardial infarction in the near term and should be hospitalized. As with all forms of angina, the ECG may not show ischemia once pain has resolved.

Coronary Artery Spasm and Transmural Ischemia

There is also a subgroup of patients who display coronary artery spasm, usually in the vicinity of an obstructive lesion but sometimes even with no occlusive coronary artery disease. Spasm may effectively produce a 100% occlusion of the affected coronary artery and can therefore cause transmural ischemia and ST elevation that is indistinguishable from that of acute myocardial infarction. For this reason, it is important to give a therapeutic trial of *nitroglycerin* to patients with ECG evidence of transmural ischemia before concluding with certainty that a myocardial infarction is in progress. Patients with transmural ischemia caused by spasm will show resolution of ST elevation when nitroglycerin is administered. Those with complete obstruction from a thrombosis will not.

Acute Myocardial Infarction

The discomfort of acute myocardial infarction (AMI) may be of the same character and location as both stable and unstable angina but is frequently more intense; that is, the discomfort is perceived as hurting more. It may come with or without exertion and is unrelieved or, at best, only partially relieved by rest or nitroglycerin.

Shortness of breath, nausea, vomiting, and diaphoresis are frequent but not necessary companions of AMI. Their presence, however, strengthens the

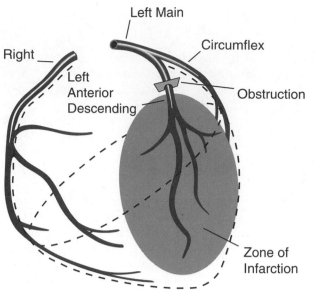

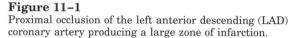

Figure 11–1
Proximal occlusion of the left anterior descending (LAD) coronary artery producing a large zone of infarction.

presumption of AMI. Particularly powerful indicators of AMI are the presence of pain in the jaws or profound diaphoresis, and chest pain patients displaying such symptoms should be considered to have myocardial infarction until proved otherwise.

Other symptoms associated with acutely diminished cardiac output may also appear with AMI, including pallor, near-syncope, and diminished mentation. Of course, sudden death resulting from ventricular fibrillation may be the presenting symptom in up to 40% of patients, although AMI is not a necessary prerequisite of ventricular fibrillation.

Pathologically, AMI is the result of complete occlusion of the coronary arterial lumen, most commonly by development of a thrombus in the diseased portion of the vessel. Muscle supplied by the affected vessel distal to the occlusion is in jeopardy of necrosis. Proximal occlusions affect a larger muscle mass than do distal occlusions (Figs. 11–1 and 11–2).

Figure 11–2
Distal occlusion of the LAD producing a much smaller zone of infarction than is seen with proximal occlusions.

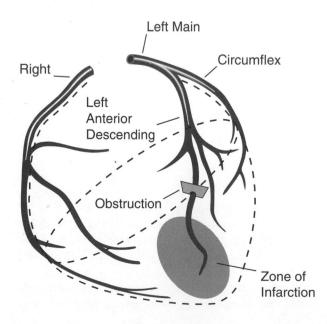

The quantity of muscle lost to necrosis in AMI is dependent upon the size of the affected vessel, the proximal or distal location of the lesion, and the quantity of collateral circulation from other vessels to the muscle in jeopardy. Loss of more than 40% of ventricular muscle in AMI generally results in cardiogenic shock and death.

You are by now familiar with the ECG changes of AMI. Remember, however, that occasionally in the early stages of either transmural or nontransmural AMI, the ECG may remain negative and not show evidence of infarction for hours. Occasionally, patients with AMI may complete their infarction and never show clear ECG evolution of AMI. This is another reason why a high index of suspicion on the basis of the patient's history is so important.

Taking the History

It is apparent from the foregoing discussion that the following are essential base line questions that must be asked of any patient with chest pain:

1. When did the discomfort begin?
2. Where do you feel it?
3. Does it travel anyplace?
4. How would you describe the discomfort?
5. Has the discomfort been constant, or does it come and go?
6. Does it feel like the discomfort you have had in the past? (For patients with documented pre-existing heart disease)
7. Is there anything that seems to aggravate the discomfort or relieve the discomfort?
8. Did you break out in a sweat, have nausea or vomiting, or become short of breath?

This list is not exhaustive, of course, but answers to these questions should be considered the minimum information necessary for an adequate history of chest pain. The questions can be asked while other tasks are being performed and should not be permitted to delay essential care or transport.

Historical factors militating against a diagnosis of ischemic heart pain include:

- Discomfort that repeatedly comes at rest but not with exercise
- Discomfort that goes away with exercise
- Discomfort on only one side of the chest but not retrosternally
- Pain that is described as "sharp"
- Pain that lasts only seconds at a time
- Pain that "flies in" and "flies out"
- Pain that lasts for hours or days at a time in the obvious absence of myocardial infarction
- Pain that is pleuritic (increases with respiration)

None of these historical factors, however, should be considered to safely rule out AMI. All of us with experience in diagnosing AMI have been misled by a history that seemed incompatible with AMI. The important factor in avoiding a missed diagnosis of AMI is to maintain a high index of suspicion.

Role of the Physical Examination

The role of the physical examination in the diagnosis of AMI should be viewed primarily as helping to lend confirmation to a diagnosis made primarily on the basis of history. It is not uncommon for the patient presenting with AMI to have an essentially normal preliminary cardiovascular examination.

Therefore, it is important not to dismiss the diagnosis of AMI or to lower the index of suspicion for AMI simply on the basis of a normal physical examination.

Findings supporting a diagnosis of AMI include pallor, cold and clammy skin, diaphoresis, and an S₄ gallop. Patients who have developed *forward failure* (low cardiac output) as a complication of AMI may also display diminished pulses, hypotension, decreased mentation, and anxiety. Signs of *backward failure* (pulmonary edema) include prominent dyspnea, jugular venous distention, use of the accessory muscles of inspiration, rales, and an S₃ gallop.

Dysrhythmias common to AMI may be discovered at the time of auscultation or may be viewed on a cardiac monitor and include ventricular ectopy, sinus bradycardia or tachycardia, atrial fibrillation, and the full spectrum of AV blocks.

Clinical Patterns of Acute Myocardial Infarction

Two major clinical categories of AMI exist, each with its own characteristic clinical pattern based on the geographic distribution of the infarction and the cardiac structures involved.

You will recall that the left coronary artery supplies the anterior wall of the left ventricle and is the principal source of blood supply to the septum and, therefore, to the bundle of His and the bundle branches.

The right coronary artery supplies the inferior or diaphragmatic portion of the left ventricle and, in most patients, supplies the sinoatrial (SA) and the atrioventricular (AV) nodes. It also supplies the right ventricle.

Anterior Wall Myocardial Infarction

Anterior myocardial infarction (MI) occurs as the result of occlusion in the distribution of the left coronary artery. It is commonly a large infarction and may be associated with sinus tachycardia, pump failure, higher degrees of heart block (Mobitz type II or third degree), or with new bundle branch block.

Higher degrees of heart block occurring with anterior MI carry a bad prognosis because they are usually the result of extensive infarction with necrosis of the ventricular septum and the bundle of His or the bundle branches. Pacing is usually required for these higher degrees of heart block but rarely alters outcome because these patients typically die of pump failure as a consequence of the extensive nature of the infarction.

Inferior Wall Myocardial Infarction

Inferior MI occurs with occlusion of the right coronary artery. It is commonly associated with a significant *vasovagal response* characterized by marked sinus bradycardia and hypotension that is usually responsive to atropine and volume expansion. Sinus bradycardia may be further aggravated by a diminution in perfusion to the SA node.

AV block when seen with inferior MI is typically lower grade (first degree or Mobitz type I) and is the result of *edema* of the AV node as opposed to necrosis. Since the level of block is in the AV node, even when block advances to third degree, there is typically a reliable junctional escape rhythm present. Pacing is not usually required, and symptomatic bradycardia can usually be adequately treated with atropine. Pump failure is less often a problem than with anterior MI, unless the patient has a more extensive than usual right coronary circulation or has lost muscle mass from a previous MI.

Patients presenting with evidence of inferior MI and isolated right heart failure (jugular venous distention and hypotension with clear lungs) should also have an ECG with leads V_3 and V_4 placed on the right side of the chest to rule out a right ventricular infarction.

Role of Serial ECGs and Continuous ST Segment Monitoring

Earlier in this chapter we discussed how the ECG may be negative in the early stages of AMI. It is often prudent in patients who have negative ECGs but a high index of suspicion for AMI to perform serial ECGs over a period of time.

Many emergency departments and coronary care units now have monitoring equipment capable of continuous ST segment monitoring. This represents the ideal ECG tool for evaluation of this category of patient because the emergency department staff becomes immediately aware of any ST segment change. In the absence of continuous ST segment monitoring, however, leaving the patient connected to the ECG machine and performing serial tracings every 10 to 15 minutes during the acute period is almost as useful.

Many hospitals have recently established chest pain evaluation centers, which incorporate approximately 6 hours of observation, serial ECGs (or continuous ST segment monitoring), and serial cardiac enzyme determinations into their evaluation of patients with chest pain of unclear etiology.

The ACLS Provider and Thrombolytic Therapy

One of the important skills of an ACLS provider is the ability to rapidly identify and prepare candidates for thrombolytic therapy. The ACLS provider can play a major role in improving the time between patient presentation and administration of thrombolytic therapy.

Pathogenesis of Acute Myocardial Infarction

In the mid 1960s, most respected pathologists held the view that acute myocardial infarction (AMI) was the result of fixed obstructive disease of the coronary arteries and that clot formation rarely played a role in AMI. In fact, at that time, the old term coronary thrombosis was dropped from the lexicon, and the familiar term myocardial infarction was substituted.

Studies performed in the 1970s and 1980s, however, confirmed that, indeed, an *acute thrombosis* occurring at the proximal end of an atherosclerotic plaque was the source of obstruction in over 85% of patients suffering AMI.[1] These studies rekindled interest in the concept of thrombolysis, ultimately resulting in a revolution in the approach to AMI.

The time required for complete necrosis of involved muscle to occur following complete coronary artery occlusion is variable and is dependent upon the presence or absence of significant *collateral circulation* and a blood pressure adequate to perfuse those collaterals. Necrosis proceeds from endocardium to epicardium (Fig. 12–1). Completion of necrosis, dependent upon the above variables, may take from 1 hour to more than 6 hours (Figs.

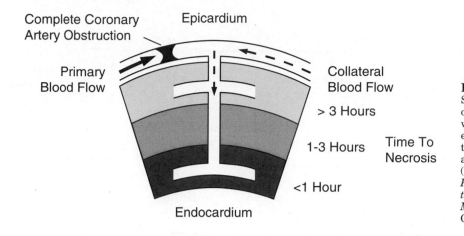

Figure 12–1
Schematic diagram showing the order of necrosis through the ventricular wall in AMI. Note that the endocardium necroses much faster than the epicardium because of less abundant collateral circulation. (Modified from Swan HJC et al.: *Practical Aspects of Thrombolysis in the Clinical Management of Acute Myocardial Infarction.* American College of Cardiology.)

12–1 and 12–2). Younger people have had fewer years over which to develop collateral circulation to ischemic areas and may necrose muscle faster than older patients. Unfortunately, an AMI in a 40-year-old may constitute the worst case of the three necrosis curves, as shown in Figure 12–2, and such a patient may lose over 1% of salvageable myocardium per minute.

Although the usual case of straightforward AMI falls within these time parameters of necrosis, there is a subgroup of patients who have what is called a *stuttering pattern* of infarction. These patients demonstrate a stuttering or intermittent pattern of pain over as long as 24 hours or more and their muscle seems to necrose more slowly than usual.

Value of Thrombolytic Agents in Acute Myocardial Infarction

The goal of thrombolytic therapy is the *reperfusion* of coronary arteries acutely occluded by a thrombus. Studies have shown that reperfusion with thrombolytic agents can result in striking reductions in mortality, in the range

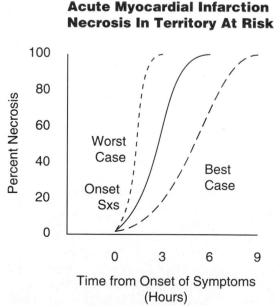

Figure 12–2
Graph depicting percent of necrosis in AMI as a function of time in the worst case, average case, and best case. Unfortunately, younger people often constitute the worst case because they have had less time than older patients to develop collateral circulation. (Modified from Swan HJC et al.: *Practical Aspects of Thrombolysis in the Clinical Management of Acute Myocardial Infarction.* American College of Cardiology.)

of 20% to 52%, with the greatest benefit being seen in those patients receiving thrombolytic therapy within 70 minutes of the onset of symptoms.[2-5] In the GISSI study, mortality was reduced by 47% if therapy was initiated within 1 hour of onset of symptoms, by 23% if within 3 hours, and by 17% if between 3 and 6 hours (Fig. 12–3).[6] More recently, other studies have suggested benefit even after 6 hours in some patients, although the reasons for this phenomenon are not entirely clear.[7-9] Some authors are recommending consideration of giving thrombolytic therapy up to 12 hours from onset of symptoms and up to 24 hours for patients with a stuttering pattern of pain.

Studies have also demonstrated improvement in *left ventricular function* following thrombolytic therapy, but these benefits are less striking than the improvement in mortality.[10]

The Early Treatment of Acute Myocardial Infarction

The advent of thrombolytic therapy has increased the importance of rapid and accurate evaluation of chest pain, including evaluation of an ECG. Unfortunately, as noted above, the benefits of therapy are exquisitely time dependent.

Most patients do not achieve maximum benefit because of delays in administration of therapy. Although in many studies patient delays in seeking care account for the single largest component of delay, events after the patient has entered the medical care system constitute the causes of delay of greatest magnitude that are potentially rapidly correctable. The average time from hospital admission to administration of thrombolytic agent in the largest multicenter studies in the United States has been almost 1½ hours, far too long to be of maximum benefit.[1]

The development of chest pain protocols that include performing an early ECG, particularly a prehospital ECG, has significantly reduced in-hospital delays. Many institutions have set a goal of administering thrombolytic therapy within 30 minutes of patient arrival, a period sometimes referred to as the *golden half hour*. One of the important skills of an ACLS provider is being adept at rapidly identifying candidates for thrombolytic therapy and preparing them for thrombolytic administration.

Figure 12–3
Percent reduction in mortality from AMI reported in the GISSI study as a function of the time from onset of symptoms to administration of a thrombolytic agent. Note that benefit of therapy drops off sharply after the first hour.

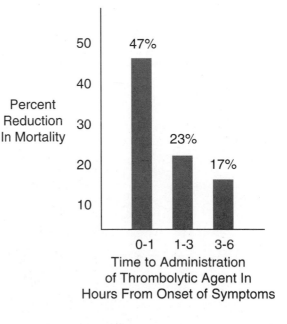

Thrombolytic Agents

Thrombolytic agents are *plasminogen activators* that convert naturally occurring plasminogen to plasmin and are able to actively dissolve, or lyse, thrombi as opposed to simply preventing thrombus propagation, as does heparin. Streptokinase, t-PA, and anisoylated plasminogen streptokinase activator complex (APSAC) are the three thrombolytic agents that have been studied in the greatest detail, although streptokinase and t-PA have enjoyed the widest use. Significant controversy has raged in the literature over their relative merits. Despite multiple studies involving tens of thousands of patients worldwide, no clear advantage has emerged for any agent. However, t-PA is much more expensive.

The theoretical advantages of t-PA in producing less of a systemic lytic state and being more "clot specific" have not translated into significantly lower rates of bleeding complications. The incidence of central nervous system bleeding has actually been slightly higher with t-PA.[8, 12–13] Streptokinase can produce allergic reactions (3.6%) or hypotensive reactions (up to 10%), but they are rarely severe.[8] Antibodies to streptokinase limit its effectiveness on a second occasion, and a previous exposure to streptokinase is an indication for the utilization of t-PA.

More important than which thrombolytic is used is how quickly it is administered.

Adjunctive Therapy

Remarkably, an aspirin, chewed immediately, augmented the reduction in mortality seen with streptokinase in the ISIS-2 study by an additional 20%.[7] In addition, aspirin reduced the incidence of nonfatal reinfarction and nonfatal stroke. Aspirin is now an integral part of clinical therapy in acute myocardial infarction and has not to date resulted in a higher incidence of bleeding.

Although still surrounded by some controversy, heparin is used by most clinicians in the post-thrombolytic period in an effort to prevent reocclusion. Heparin administered simultaneously with t-PA has improved t-PA reperfusion rates.[13]

There is no contraindication to using other traditional therapies during thrombolytic therapy, including nitroglycerin, beta blockers, calcium channel antagonists, and antiarrhythmics.

Reperfusion

Reperfusion following thrombolytic therapy may be manifested by prompt relief of pain, decrease in ST segment elevation, reperfusion arrhythmias, early "washout" of enzymes, and occasionally signs of improved left ventricular function. Reperfusion dysrhythmias, which may include both atrial and ventricular ectopy, are usually short-lived and rarely require treatment. An accelerated idioventricular rhythm is particularly common. Nevertheless, continuous monitoring during thrombolytic therapy is imperative.

Time to reperfusion is highly variable, ranging from 5 minutes to 2 or 3 hours, but most patients reperfuse within the first hour. The incidence of reperfusion as a result of intravenous thrombolytic therapy is generally accepted to be over 70% and in some studies has exceeded 90%.

Reperfusion is usually accompanied by resolution of ST segment elevation in cases that reperfuse early. Figure 12–4A is the tracing of a 59-year-old white male with acute inferior wall myocardial infarction taken at 9:23 AM during administration of streptokinase. Figure 12–4B is from the same patient taken 7 minutes later at 9:30 AM after sudden relief of pain. Note that substantial resolution of both ST segment elevation and reciprocal depression has occurred with reperfusion. Late reperfusion, after substantial necrosis has occurred, is less likely to produce resolution of ECG changes.

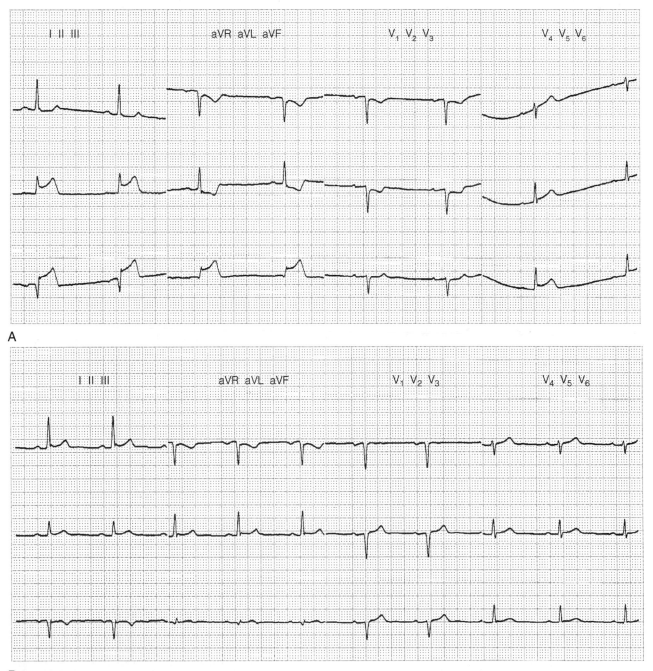

Figure 12–4. *A.* Tracing from a 59-year-old white male taken at 9:23 AM during streptokinase administration for acute inferior wall MI. Note typical prominent ST elevation in the inferior wall with reciprocal depression in leads I, aVL, and V_1 and V_2. *B.* Second tracing taken from the same patient 7 minutes later at 9:30 AM after sudden relief of pain. Note substantial resolution of ST segment elevation and reciprocal depression that has occurred with reperfusion.

Complications of Therapy

The most significant adverse reaction of thrombolytic therapy is, of course, bleeding. Intracranial bleeding is the most serious complication (<1%), but in actuality it represents approximately the same incidence of stroke as occurs in control groups with AMI.[14] The overall incidence of bleeding is less than 5% when patients with uncontrolled hypertension and cerebrovascular disease are excluded. Nevertheless, special measures are warranted in the care of patients undergoing thrombolysis to reduce exogenous stimuli to bleeding, such as needlesticks and invasive procedures.

Dosing t-PA on the basis of body weight has reduced the incidence of bleeding with t-PA.

Contraindications

As the relative safety and efficacy of thrombolytic therapy have become more clearly established, the number of absolute and relative contraindications has diminished. Age, for example, is no longer an obstacle to therapy. In the ISIS-2 study, patients as old as 90 years were treated, and there was a 32% mortality reduction with thrombolysis among patients in the over-70 age group.[7]

Absolute Contraindications

- Active or recent gastrointestinal bleed or ulcer
- History of cerebrovascular accident in last 6 months
- Recent intracranial surgery or trauma
- Intracranial neoplasm; arteriovenous malformation
- Known bleeding diathesis
- Severe, uncontrolled hypertension > 200/110

Relative Contraindications

- Recent (10 days) major surgery
- Recent (10 days) gastrointestinal or genitourinary surgery
- Recent (10 days) trauma
- Cardiopulmonary resuscitation of > 10 minutes
- Blood pressure > 180/110
- Infected heart valves (infectious endocarditis)
- Acute pericarditis
- Hemostatic defects
- Pregnancy
- History of a bleeding condition in the eye
- Currently on anticoagulants (sodium warfarin, Coumadin)

Some authors also exclude patients with pulmonary edema or in cardiogenic shock (Killip classes III and IV—Fig. 12–5) from consideration for thrombolytic therapy because of the absence of statistically significant benefit from thrombolysis in this group of patients. Mortality rates in cardiogenic shock have been more positively affected by emergency coronary angioplasty (PTCA).[15] Nevertheless, the presence of pulmonary edema or cardiogenic shock should not be considered a contraindication.

Class I	No clinical heart failure.
Class II	Rales 1/2 way up lung fields.
Class III	Rales in all lung fields (pulmonary edema).
Class IV	Cardiogenic shock; BP < 90 systolic; pulmonary edema.

Figure 12–5
The Killip classification system of clinical heart failure.

Identifying Candidates for Thrombolysis

Potential candidates for thrombolytic therapy include:

- Patients of any age
- Patients with a history compatible with AMI
- Patients with pain of less than 12 hours' duration
- Patients with an ECG compatible with AMI
- No resolution of pain and ST segment elevation with nitroglycerin administration
- Patients who have no absolute contraindications

It is not necessary or even desirable to confirm AMI with enzyme determinations. Indeed, reliance on laboratory testing for confirmation of diagnosis is one of the causes of unnecessary delays in administration of therapy.

ECG criteria for compatibility with AMI should include ST elevation of 1 mm or greater in at least two contiguous (adjacent) limb leads or elevation of 2 mm or greater in at least two contiguous precordial leads.

You learned in Chapter 9 that the changes of left bundle branch block (LBBB) can simulate but can also mask an acute anterior myocardial infarction. For this reason, patients presenting with LBBB and a history compatible with AMI should be strongly considered for thrombolytic therapy.

Finally, you have also learned that ST elevation is evanescent; that is, it comes and goes. Patients may present with Q waves and T wave inversion after the ST elevation has resolved and still be within the required time frames for administration of thrombolytic agents.

In summary, patients with the following ECG criteria should be considered for thrombolytic therapy:

1. ST elevation 1 mm or greater in two contiguous limb leads
2. ST elevation 2 mm or greater in two contiguous precordial leads
3. LBBB, particularly if new
4. New pathologic Q waves and T wave inversion

Remember that in order to avoid a mistaken diagnosis of AMI with each of these ECG criteria, it is important to have a history compatible with AMI. In addition, in order to avoid administering thrombolytics to patients who have transmural ischemia and ST segment elevation on the basis of coronary artery spasm alone, it is important to administer a brief therapeutic trial of nitroglycerin before concluding that the patient has an AMI.

Components of Delay in Thrombolysis

The total elapsed time from the onset of symptoms to administration of a thrombolytic agent can be divided into three distinct phases. The first phase is the time required for the patient to recognize that something is wrong and make the decision to access the medical system. The second is the time required for the prehospital emergency medical system to respond, render emergency care, and transport the patient to a medical facility. The third phase consists of the time required for the hospital to recognize AMI, qualify the patient, and administer the thrombolytic agent.

Phase 1 is beyond the direct control of medical personnel. Efforts to impact the first phase through programs of public education have been disappointing. The second and third phases, however, are within the direct control of the medical community. Reducing times to thrombolysis requires a coordinated effort between prehospital and hospital personnel and the establishment of clear protocols for the evaluation and treatment of patients with chest pain.

Reducing Times to Thrombolysis

Prehospital Protocols

The effort to speed the administration of thrombolytic agents should begin with the prehospital emergency medical system. Multiple studies have now clearly demonstrated that in-hospital times to thrombolysis are significantly reduced by the performance of a prehospital ECG.[11, 16–19] Prehospital ACLS providers have readily mastered the technique of performing an ECG, and on-scene times have been minimally affected by this additional task, being increased by only 2 to 5 minutes.

Interpretation of the ECG can be accomplished via cellular telemetry by a physician at the base hospital, by computer interpretation, or by independent sight-reading of the tracing by trained prehospital ACLS providers. The hospital emergency department is then notified by radio that a prequalified potential candidate for thrombolysis is en route. The ability of the hospital team to "gear up" based on such field reports has been reported to save from 29 to 71 minutes in-hospital.[16–19]

Other necessary but time-consuming elements of every thrombolytic protocol, such as drawing blood, starting three intravenous lines, and administering aspirin, can also often be partially or completely accomplished en route. Finally, the prehospital provider can also continue to converse with the patient during the above procedures and complete the initial screen for contraindications to thrombolysis. Figure 12–6 shows one example of a field-tested prehospital protocol that has been proven to be practical.

Note that when the ECG is negative but the history is compatible with AMI, the patient is placed in a category of "high index of suspicion" that warrants continuation of the protocol and serial ECGs.

In-Hospital Protocols

Elapsed times from patient arrival to initiation of thrombolytic therapy at the hospital cannot be reduced without two key hospital policies that have been agreed upon by the medical staff. The first is that hospital emergency department physicians must have the ability to initiate thrombolytic therapy on their own authority. Waiting for an evaluation by a consulting cardiologist is one of the biggest sources of in-hospital delay.

The second key policy is that thrombolytic therapy must be initiated in the emergency department as opposed to being delayed until the patient is transferred to the coronary care unit.

With these two key policies in place, the emergency department can proceed to establish effective protocols for speeding thrombolysis.

WAYNESBORO HOSPITAL - MEDIC 2
PREHOSPITAL CHEST PAIN PROTOCOL

Patient Name _____   ALS Provider _____

Date _____   Time Onset of Pain _____

Trip # _____

Y or N

_____ 1. HISTORY compatible with acute MI?

_____ 2. PHYSICAL exam compatible with acute MI?

_____ 3. INITIAL THERAPY as indicated.

_____ 4. ELECTROCARDIOGRAPHIC CHANGES compatible with acute MI?

_____ 5. CONTRAINDICATIONS to thrombolytic therapy?

        ABSOLUTE (Check only those with a *positive* history)

        _____ a) Active internal bleeding
        _____ b) History of cerebrovascular accident
        _____ c) Recent (within 2 months) intracranial or intraspinal surgery or trauma
        _____ d) Intracranial neoplasm, arteriovenous malformation, or aneurysm
        _____ e) Known bleeding diathesis
        _____ f) Severe, uncontrolled hypertension (>210/120)

        RELATIVE
        _____ a) Recent (10 days) major surgery
        _____ b) Recent (10 days) GI or GU bleeding
        _____ c) Recent (10 days) trauma (including CPR)
        _____ d) BP >180/110
        _____ e) Infected heart valves
        _____ f) Acute pericarditis
        _____ g) Hemostatic defects
        _____ h) Pregnant
        _____ i) Over 75 years of age
        _____ j) History of bleeding condition in eye (diabetic retinopathy)
        _____ k) Currently on anticoagulants (Coumadin)
        _____ l) History of previous thrombolytic therapy with strep

_____ 6. THROMBOLYTIC THERAPY INDICATED in Provider's opinion?   TIME of decision:_____

_____ 7. IF NO, IS INDEX OF SUSPICION still high enough to proceed with protocol?

_____ 8. CONTACT MED COMMAND
        _____ a) Give report
        _____ b) Include verbal evaluation of EKG
        _____ c) Request approval for thrombolytic protocol if indicated

_____ 9. APPROVAL RECEIVED for thrombolytic protocol from Med Commander?

==

_____ 10. SECOND IV D5/W with Twin-cath (Leave all unsuccessful IV's in place, tightly taped)

_____ 11. DRAW BLOODS when starting IV

_____ 12. ADMINISTER ASPIRIN 325 MG if ordered by Med Commander. Check for *ASPIRIN ALLERGY*.

Figure 12–6. Sample prehospital chest pain protocol that includes performance of a 12-lead ECG.

Emergency department protocols for dealing with potential thrombolytic candidates should be the equivalent of a major trauma plan and should carry the same sense of urgency. The following are essential components of an effective protocol:

1. The protocol must be in writing, including drug preparation instructions and dosage charts, and must be conveniently posted in appropriate locations.
2. Nursing triage staff must have the ability to initiate the protocol before the patient has been seen by the physician, including starting intravenous lines, drawing blood, and performing a 12-lead ECG, particularly on patients who do not arrive via the emergency medical system.
3. All necessary supplies and medications for thrombolytic therapy should be kept in a kit or at a single readily accessible location.
4. Minimum mandatory criteria necessary for emergency department physicians to initiate thrombolytic therapy should be confined to a history and ECG compatible with AMI. Therapy should not be delayed while staff awaits laboratory results.

The goal of such organizational efforts should be to administer thrombolytic therapy to appropriate candidates within less than 30 minutes from the time of their arrival in the emergency department. A few institutions have been successful in routinely accomplishing initiation of therapy in less than 15 minutes when the presentation of AMI is straightforward.

REFERENCES

1. DeWood MA, Spores J, Notske R et al. Prevalence of total coronary artery occlusion during the early hours of transmural myocardial infarction. *N Engl J Med* 1980;303:897–902.
2. Cerqueirs M, Litwin P, Martin J et al. Infarct size reduction and preservation of ejection fractions with very early thrombolytic treatment for myocardial infarction: radionuclide results from the Myocardial Infarction Triage and Intervention Trial. *Circulation* 1992;86(suppl 1):643. Abstract.
3. GISSI: Longterm effects of intravenous thrombolysis in acute myocardial infarction: a final report of the GISSI study. *Lancet* 1987;2:871–874.
4. Koren G, Weiss AT, Hasin Y et al. Prevention of myocardial damage in acute myocardial ischemia by early treatment with intravenous streptokinase. *N Engl J Med* 1985;313: 1384–1389.
5. Fine DG, Weiss AT, Sapoznikov D et al: Importance of early initiation of intravenous streptokinase therapy for acute myocardial infarction. *Am J Cardiol* 1986;58:411–417.
6. Italian Group for the Study of Streptokinase in Myocardial Infarction (GISSI): Effectiveness of intravenous thrombolytic treatment in acute myocardial infarction. *Lancet* 1986;1:397.
7. ISIS-2 (Second International Study of Infarct Survival) Collaborative Group: Randomized trial of intravenous streptokinase, oral aspirin, both, or neither among 17,187 cases of suspected acute myocardial infarction. *Lancet* 1988;2(8607):349–360.
8. ISIS-3 (Third International Study of Infarct Survival) Collaborative Group: A randomized comparison of streptokinase vs tissue plasminogen activator vs anistreplase and of aspirin plus heparin vs aspirin alone among 41,299 cases of suspected acute myocardial infarction. *Lancet* 1992;339(8796):753–770.
9. LATE Study Group: Late Assessment of Thrombolytic Efficacy (LATE) study with alteplase 6–24 hours after onset of acute myocardial infarction. *Lancet* 1993;342(8874):759–766.
10. Tiefenbrunn AJ, Sobel BE: The impact of coronary thrombolysis on myocardial infarction. *Fibrinolysis* 1989;3:1–15.
11. Kereiakes DJ, Weaver WD, Anderson JL et al. Time delays in the diagnosis and treatment of acute myocardial infarction: a tale of eight cities. Report from the PreHospital Study Group and the Cincinnati Heart Project. *Am Heart J* 1990;120:773–780.
12. GISSI-2: A factorial randomized trial of alteplase versus streptokinase and heparin versus no heparin among 12,490 patients with acute myocardial infarction. *Lancet* 1990;336:65–71.
13. GUSTO: An international randomized trial comparing four thrombolytic strategies for acute myocardial infarction. *N Engl J Med* 1993;329(10):723–725.
14. Tiefenbrunn AJ, Ludbrook PA: Coronary thrombolysis—it's worth the risk. *JAMA* 1989;261:2107.
15. Lange RA, Hillis LD: Immediate angioplasty for acute myocardial infarction. *N Engl J Med* 1993;328(10):726–728.

16. Karagounis L, Ipsen SK, Jessop MR et al. Impact of field-transmitted electrocardiography on time to in-hospital thrombolytic therapy in acute myocardial infarction. *Am J Cardiol* 1990;66:786–791.
17. Gibler WB, Kereiakes DJ, Dean EN et al. Prehospital diagnosis and treatment of acute myocardial infarction: a North-South perspective. *Am Heart J* 1991;121:1–11.
18. Kennedy JW, Weaver WD: The potential for prehospital thrombolytic therapy. *Clin Cardiol* 1990;13(Suppl 8):VIII23–26.
19. Foster DB, Dufendach JH, Barkdoll CM et al. Prehospital recognition of AMI using independent nurse/paramedic 12-lead ECG evaluation: impact on in-hospital times to thrombolysis in a rural community hospital. *Am J Emerg Med* 1994;1:25–31.

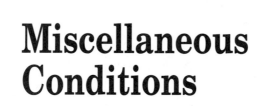

CHAPTER
13

Miscellaneous Conditions

$\mathbf{I}$n this chapter, I discuss a potpourri of essentially unrelated medical conditions that can sometimes produce dramatic changes in the appearance of the ECG.

Electrolyte Disturbances

Alterations in certain serum electrolytes, particularly in serum potassium and calcium, can produce rather dramatic changes in the ECG because of the roles of electrolytes in membrane repolarization and depolarization. As you will recall, influx and efflux of positive ions across cell membranes are the basis for the electrical activity of cells. Alterations in electrolyte concentrations could be expected to change the behavior of that electrical activity and therefore to also change the ECG.

Hypokalemia

When serum potassium concentrations fall below about 3.0 mEq/L, ST segments begin to sag, T waves begin to flatten or invert, and U waves begin to become more prominent, sometimes exceeding the T wave in height. Often, the flattened T wave and the prominent U wave begin to merge, giving the false appearance of a prolonged QT interval.

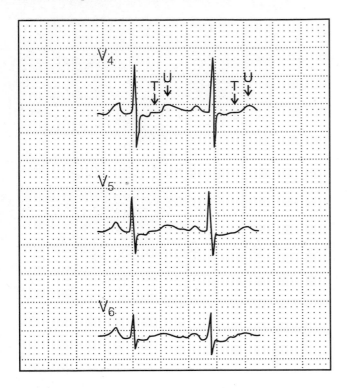

Figure 13–1
Leads V$_4$ through V$_6$ from a patient with a serum
potassium of 2.6. Note J-point depression and a sagging
ST segment. The flattened T waves and prominent U
waves have almost merged to give the false appearance of
a prolonged QT interval.

Figure 13–1 illustrates these hallmarks of hypokalemia. Note that the
take-off, or J-point, of the ST segment is depressed. The net effect of these
changes is a rather undulating appearance in the combined ST segment, T
wave, and U wave.

Patients with hypokalemia are more prone to life-threatening ventricular
dysrhythmias, particularly when taking digitalis preparations. Common factors predisposing to hypokalemia include diuretic administration and vomiting
(hypochloremic alkalosis), and correction of diabetic ketoacidosis without adequate potassium replacement.

Hyperkalemia

Many of the ECG changes seen with hyperkalemia are simply the opposite
of those seen with hypokalemia. As serum potassium levels begin to rise above
about 5.5 mEq/L, T waves become very tall and peaked (Fig. 13–2). J-point
ST elevation may occur, simulating acute myocardial infarction. Further elevations in potassium begin to produce lengthening PR intervals and nonspecific,
but often dramatic, QRS widening. P waves begin to flatten and may disappear
altogether. The terminal event is asystole or ventricular fibrillation.

Figure 13–3A is the ECG of a 52-year-old white male seen in the emergency
department with a serum potassium level of 8.1 mEq/L on the basis of renal
failure and diabetic ketoacidosis. Note that P waves cannot be seen in most
leads, and there is diffuse nonspecific widening of the QRS to over .20 second.
Figure 13–3B is a tracing taken on the same patient after treatment with
intravenous calcium gluconate, bicarbonate, and insulin. Note that although
clear P waves have not yet returned, the QRS has dramatically narrowed, and
T waves in leads V$_4$ and V$_5$ have taken on the tall, peaked appearance typical
of lower levels of hyperkalemia.

As with hypokalemia, ventricular fibrillation may be the ultimate consequence of progressive hyperkalemia. Common causes of hyperkalemia include
renal failure, acidosis, administration of aldosterone antagonists, and administration of exogenous potassium.

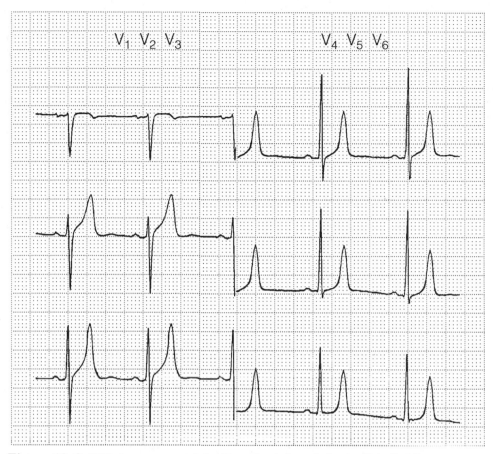

Figure 13–2. ECG changes associated with moderate hyperkalemia. Note that T waves are tall and symmetrically peaked and that there is mild J-point elevation in V_2 and V_3.

Hypocalcemia

The hallmark of hypocalcemia is a prolonged QT interval. Occasionally T wave inversion will also occur, but this is unusual. Clinically significant hypocalcemia is rare, and the primary cause is usually hypoparathyroidism.

Hypercalcemia

Elevations of serum calcium produce changes opposite to those produced by hypocalcemia, namely a shortened QT interval, often with a very abrupt upslope of the T wave.

Hypercalcemia is more common than hypocalcemia. Major causes include advanced malignancy, hyperparathyroidism, and sarcoidosis.

Drug-Induced ECG Changes

A number of drugs can produce changes in the ECG, but the most important are digitalis, quinidine, and procainamide. The changes induced by these drugs, although sometimes characteristic, are often nonspecific and easily confused with other causes of ECG abnormalities.

The primary usefulness of recognizing the abnormalities that can be caused by drugs is in ruling out a drug-induced etiology for various ECG findings before concluding that the changes are the result of primary myocardial disease.

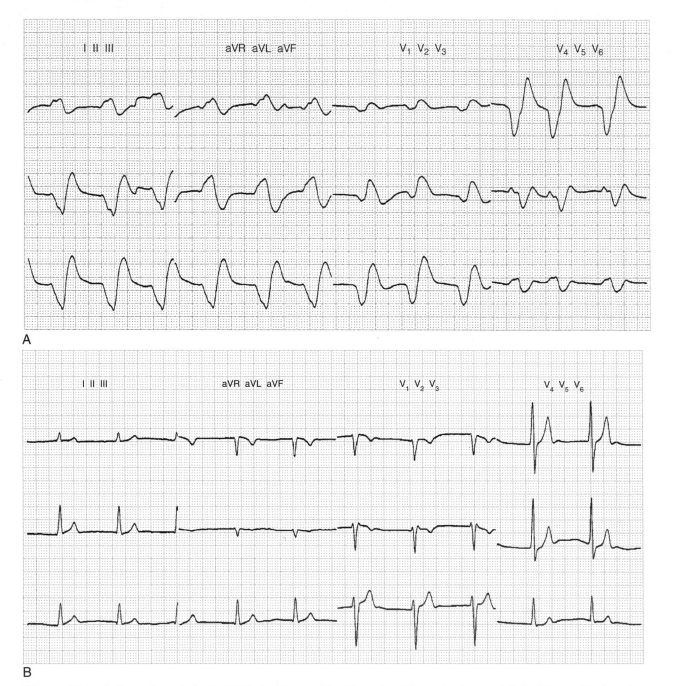

Figure 13–3. *A.* Severe hyperkalemia. ECG of a 52-year-old white male with renal failure and diabetic ketoacidosis and a serum potassium of 8.1. P waves are visible only in leads V_5 and V_6, and the QRS is widened to over .20 second. *B.* ECG of the same patient as in *A* after treatment with IV calcium gluconate, insulin, and sodium bicarbonate.

In addition, a familiarity with drug-induced ECG changes can aid in suspecting drug toxicity when ECG changes occur acutely in patients on these drugs.

Digitalis Effect

Digitalis products, even in therapeutic, nontoxic doses, can produce sagging of the ST segment, flattening of T waves, and shortening of the QT interval. The ST depression in digitalis toxicity is upwardly concave, as opposed to its appearance in left ventricular hypertrophy, for instance, where it is upwardly

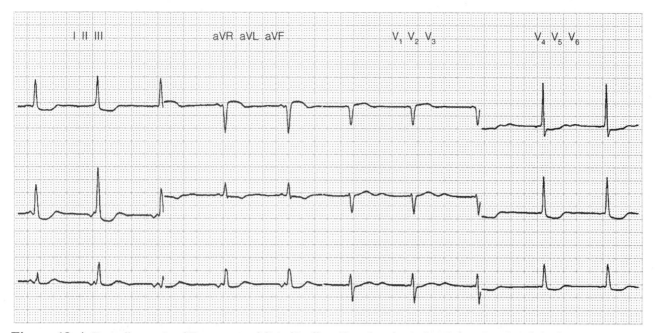

Figure 13–4. Typically sagging ST segments of digitalis effect. Note that the patient is in a junctional rhythm.

convex. Figure 13–4 shows these typical changes in the ECG of a patient with therapeutic levels of digoxin.

Digitalis intoxication can produce multiple rhythm disturbances, including the classic junctional tachycardia, paroxysmal atrial tachycardia with block, all forms of ventricular ectopy, and all forms of heart block.

Quinidine Effect

The primary effect of quinidine is on T waves and the QT interval. T waves become widened, flattened, and ultimately inverted. Marked lengthening of the QT interval can occur and can contribute to the pro-arrhythmic effect sometimes noted with quinidine. In addition, significant widening of the QRS occurs at toxic levels.

Figure 13–5 shows the precordial leads of a 75-year-old white female who had recently been started on quinidine for atrial fibrillation. This tracing was taken just minutes after conversion from an episode of ventricular fibrillation precipitated by the pro-arrhythmic effect of quinidine. Note that the QT interval is prolonged and that the T waves are flattened and widened.

Procainamide Effect

The primary effect of procainamide is widening of the QRS at toxic doses. An increase in QRS duration of 50% or more is one of the end points of procainamide administration.

Intracranial Hemorrhage

Cerebral hemorrhage or other causes of a rapid rise in intracranial pressure can produce bradycardia, widening of the T waves, and T wave inversion across the precordial leads. Such changes are an ominous prognostic sign. Figure 13–6 shows the tracing of an elderly white female with an ultimately fatal extensive cerebral hemorrhage.

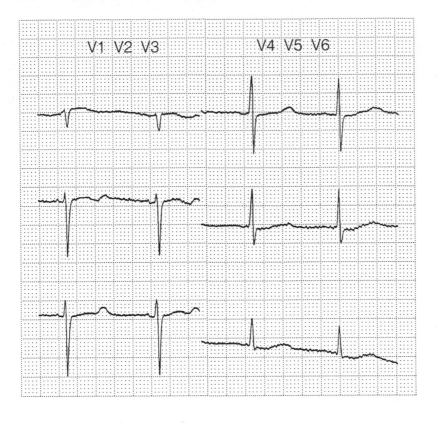

Figure 13–5
Precordial leads of a 75-year-old white female taking quinidine. Tracing was taken just after DC countershock for ventricular fibrillation. Note the prolonged QT interval and flattening and widening of T waves. Considerable muscle artifact is present.

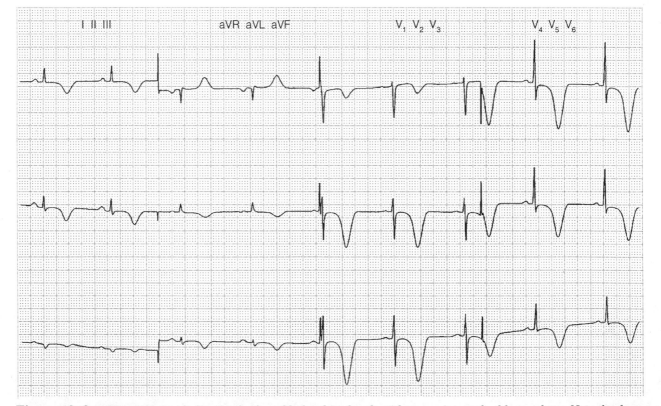

Figure 13–6. ECG tracing just before death of an elderly white female with a massive cerebral hemorrhage. Note the deep symmetrical T wave inversion, particularly across the precordial leads.

Diffuse Low Voltage

Low voltage throughout the 12-lead ECG can be seen with hypothyroidism, pericardial effusion, and diffuse cardiomyopathy of ischemic or other origin.

Pericarditis

The ECG changes of acute pericarditis, like those of acute myocardial infarction, go through an evolutionary process over a period of weeks. But, as you will recall from the discussion of the differential diagnosis of ST elevation in Chapter 9, there are significant differences that usually permit us to distinguish between the two.

ST elevation is the usual initial hallmark of both pericarditis and acute myocardial infarction. The ST elevation of pericarditis, however, is usually upwardly concave, widespread throughout all leads, and without reciprocal ST depression.

T wave inversion follows ST elevation as the ST segments return to base line, but the Q waves seen with acute myocardial infarction never develop.

Another interesting and unique finding with pericarditis is depression of the PR segment. Figure 13–7 is the ECG of a 37-year-old white male with acute viral pericarditis. Note that the PR segments are depressed below the base line and that there is widespread upwardly concave ST elevation, without reciprocal depression and without Q wave formation.

Acute pericarditis often undergoes ECG evolution, much as does acute myocardial infarction, except for Q wave formation, which does not occur with pericarditis. ST segment elevation will show resolution, however, and, as with acute myocardial infarction, T waves may invert.

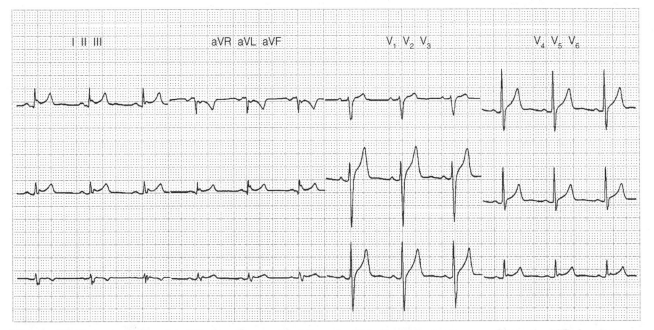

Figure 13–7. Acute viral pericarditis in a 37-year-old white male Note the widespread, upwardly concave ST elevation, depressed PR segment, and absence of Q waves or reciprocal depression.

Wolff-Parkinson-White Syndrome

Wolff-Parkinson-White (WPW) syndrome is the result of a congenital *accessory pathway* to the ventricles that bypasses the atrioventricular (AV) node, resulting in *pre-excitation* of the ventricles. The impulse still goes down through the AV node normally but also goes down the accessory pathway, which conducts much faster than does the AV node. The result is that the impulse gets to the ventricles early via the accessory pathway, producing an early slurred upstroke of the R wave, called a *delta wave* (see Fig. 2–4).

This early delta wave also produces a short PR interval and widening of the QRS. Often, however, the remainder of the QRS after the delta wave looks normal because, in many instances, most of the ventricular muscle is still depolarized via the normal conduction system. In other cases, a large amount of muscle may be depolarized by slow muscle-to-muscle conduction initiated by the accessory pathway and may produce a QRS, an ST segment, and T waves looking more like a bundle branch block pattern.

Figure 13–8 is the tracing of a 44-year-old white male with a history of WPW syndrome. Note that the PR interval is short and there is a clear delta wave seen in most, but not all, leads. In the case of this particular patient, the remainder of the QRS looks normal.

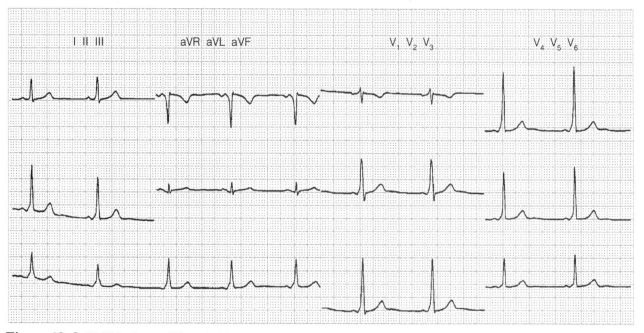

Figure 13–8. Wolff-Parkinson-White (WPW) syndrome with a short PR interval and delta waves seen in most leads.

Appendix 1

Case Presentations

This section is designed to give you some practice in implementing your new-found knowledge in making clinical decisions regarding the patient with chest pain, much as ACLS megacodes permit you to practice resuscitation. There are ten practice case presentations. You will have the opportunity to make decisions in a sequential fashion, much as you would in real-life clinical situations. Sometimes you will be functioning in the prehospital environment, and sometimes in the emergency department or coronary care unit. For purposes of this section you should assume that the phrase *prehospital thrombolytic protocol* refers to (1) starting three IV lines (one single lumen line and one twin-catheter line), (2) drawing blood specimens for laboratory analysis in the process, and (3) administering one aspirin to be chewed—all of these in preparation for thrombolysis in the emergency department. The phrase does *not* imply administering thrombolytics in the field.

Policies regarding the authority of individual paramedics, nurses, and even physicians to initiate procedures or therapy vary from jurisdiction to jurisdiction. Assume for the purposes of this section that you always have the authority to proceed without consulting a higher authority when presented with diagnostic or therapeutic options. You should find it fun.

CASE NUMBER 1

You are functioning as a prehospital ALS provider today. You are dispatched to a local accounting firm to help a 39-year-old black male with a chief complaint of retrosternal chest discomfort with minimal radiation to the left shoulder. The pain came on while he was sitting at his desk, is described as a pressure, and has been present for a little over 3 hours. He admits to mild nausea but denies vomiting, diaphoresis, or shortness of breath. He has not tried antacids or nitroglycerin for relief. He awoke with a similar discomfort about three nights ago, went into the bathroom and got a drink, then lay down and fell asleep again. He has had no exertional chest discomfort with exercise such as mowing the lawn with a push lawnmower.

He has been told in the past that he has "a little" high blood pressure, but no medications were prescribed. He smokes one pack of cigarettes daily. His father died in his early fifties quite suddenly.

Physical examination reveals a mildly obese black male who appears anxious. Pulse, 80. Respirations, 20. BP, 184/112. His skin is warm and dry. He has no jugular venous distention. The lungs are clear. Heart rhythm is regular, and the heart tones are not muffled. He has no peripheral edema.

1. With regard to the pain, you conclude that
    a) the history is sufficient to be compatible with AMI (acute myocardial infarction).
    b) the history is not compatible with AMI.

2. With regard to the physical examination, you conclude that
    a) the physical examination lends support to the diagnosis of AMI.
    b) the physical examination neither confirms nor denies the possibility of AMI.

3. Your first procedural step should be to
   a) give sublingual nitroglycerin, 0.4 mg.
   b) start a medical IV, attach the patient to a cardiac monitor, start O_2.
   c) perform a 12-lead electrocardiogram.
   d) question the patient regarding contraindications to thrombolytic therapy.

4. Your second procedural step should be to
   a) give sublingual nitroglycerin, 0.4 mg.
   b) start a medical IV, attach the patient to a cardiac monitor, start O_2.
   c) perform a 12-lead electrocardiogram.
   d) question the patient regarding contraindications to thrombolytic therapy.

5. Your third procedural step should be to
   a) give sublingual nitroglycerin, 0.4 mg.
   b) start a medical IV, attach the patient to a cardiac monitor, start O_2.
   c) perform a 12-lead electrocardiogram.
   d) question the patient regarding contraindications to thrombolytic therapy.

You have performed a 12-lead ECG (see Appendix Figure 1). Questioning conducted during performance of the ECG revealed that the patient had a hernia repair 2 years ago. He admits to an allergy to aspirin and states that he breaks out in hives when he takes the drug.

6. Upon completion of the ECG, you quickly note that the patient's electrocardiogram shows
   a) a normal axis.
   b) right axis deviation.
   c) left axis deviation.
   d) an indeterminate axis.

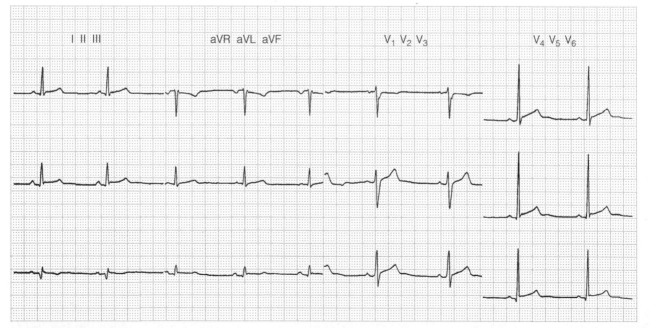

Appendix Figure 1

7. With regard to contraindications to aspirin, you conclude that
    a) contraindications exist.
    b) no contraindications exist.

8. With regard to contraindications to thrombolytic agents, on the basis of currently available information you conclude that
    a) absolute contraindications exist.
    b) relative contraindications exist.
    c) no contraindications exist.

The patient reports no relief after a single spray of nitroglycerin into the buccal mucosa.

9. Upon contacting medical command by radio you report that the ECG shows
    a) an acute inferior myocardial infarction.
    b) an acute anterior MI.
    c) an inferior MI that may be old.
    d) an anterior MI that may be old.
    e) benign early repolarization changes.
    f) a left bundle branch block simulating anterior MI.
    g) acute periocarditis.
    h) a normal ECG.
    i) nonspecific ST changes.

10. Your field assessment, as reported to medical command, is that
    a) sufficient evidence of AMI exists to recommend thrombolytic therapy and to institute the prehospital thrombolytic protocol, with the exception of aspirin.
    b) sufficient evidence of AMI exists to recommend thrombolytic therapy, with the exception of aspirin, if relative contraindications can be removed.
    c) evidence of AMI exists, but absolute contraindications prohibit thrombolytic therapy.
    d) evidence of AMI exists, but relative contraindications rule out thrombolytic therapy.
    e) insufficient evidence of AMI exists to recommend either thrombolytic therapy or implementation of the prehospital thrombolytic protocol.
    f) insufficient evidence of AMI exists to recommend thrombolytic therapy at present, but the index of suspicion is still high enough to warrant implementation of the prehospital thrombolytic protocol, with the exception of aspirin.

ANSWERS AND CASE DISCUSSION

1.a 2.b 3.b 4.c 5.a 6.a 7.a 8.b 9.e 10.f

This 39-year-old man had the significant risk factors of a family history of cardiovascular disease, cigarette smoking, and hypertension. Although vomiting, diaphoresis, and shortness of breath were not present, his history is still compatible with AMI. The physical examination is not helpful in this instance and neither confirms nor denies the possibility of AMI. As always, the first steps to be taken should be those that are necessary to protect the patient's life should an adverse event such as ventricular fibrillation occur. Therefore, starting an IV, monitoring the patient, and starting O_2 are the first steps.

Because administration of nitroglycerin could cause resolution of important diagnostic changes on the ECG, such as ST elevation or depression, the ECG should be performed before nitroglycerin is administered. Little harm is done by delaying nitroglycerin for the several minutes required to do the ECG, and you may prevent the patient from facing the possibility of an inconclusive diagnosis that would have been clear if the ECG had been done first.

The ECG tracing shows a normal axis of about 30°. ST elevation, which is upwardly concave, is widespread in all walls of the heart. There is no reciprocal depression. A small Q is present in lead III, but it is not pathologic, and there is no pathologic Q present in adjacent lead aVF. There is no PR segment depression, as is often seen in pericarditis. Therefore, benign early repolarization changes are the most likely source of the ST elevation, although pericarditis is still possible.

The patient's current hypertension provides a relative contraindication to thrombolytic agents, although one could still be administered if the projected benefit outweighed the risk, or if treatment was administered and resulted in the BP falling below 180/110. Aspirin is, of course, absolutely contraindicated because of the clear history of allergy.

We are thus left with a patient with significant risk factors and a history compatible with AMI, who has a contraindication to aspirin and a relative contraindication to thrombolytics. His ECG is not compatible with AMI at the present time. Nonetheless, his history is compatible with AMI, and it is quite possible that a repeat ECG upon arrival at the hospital might show AMI. Therefore, there is insufficient evidence of AMI to recommend him for thrombolytic therapy, but it is probably best to place him in a category of "negative ECG, but high index of suspicion" and go ahead and draw blood and start three IVs while en route to the hospital.

CASE NUMBER 2

You are functioning for Case 2 as an emergency department physician. It is 10:15 PM. The nurses ask you to see a 52-year-old white female with a chief complaint of epigastric and lower retrosternal "indigestion" that radiates through to between her shoulderblades. The pain came on about 6:45 PM, shortly after a supper of ham and potatoes. She has never had a similar pain. She admits to nausea, and vomited one time shortly after dinner. Her blouse became damp with perspiration after vomiting. She feels mildly short of breath. She tried a half teaspoon of baking soda in half a glass of water to relieve the indigestion but got no relief.

The patient carries a history of hypertension and diabetes. She is taking metoprolol 50 mg bid, and an oral hypoglycemic. There is no history of tobacco use. She has no knowledge of what her cholesterol level might be. Her father died of a stroke in his 70s, and her mother died of heart failure also in her 70s, but she can think of no one in the family who ever had a heart attack.

Physical examination reveals an obese white female who appears uncomfortable. Pulse, 75. Respirations, 22. BP, 190/114. Her skin is warm but damp. She has no jugular venous distention. The lungs are clear. Heart rhythm is regular, and an S4 gallop is audible. Her abdomen is soft and not really tender, but it makes her feel sick at the stomach when you palpate the epigastrium. She has no peripheral edema.

1. With regard to the pain, you conclude that
   a) the history is adequate to be compatible with AMI (acute myocardial infarction).
   b) the history is not compatible with AMI.

2. With regard to the physical examination, you conclude that
   a) the physical examination lends support to the diagnosis of AMI.
   b) the physical examination neither confirms nor denies the possibility of AMI.

The nursing staff has already started O$_2$ at 4 liters by nasal cannula and has attached the patient to the cardiac monitor, noninvasive BP machine, and pulse oximeter.

3. Your first procedural step should be to
   a) order sublingual nitroglycerin, 0.4 mg.
   b) order a medical IV.
   c) perform a stat 12-lead electrocardiogram.
   d) order the appropriate bloodwork.
   e) order a gallbladder sonogram.

4. Your second procedural step should be to
   a) order sublingual nitroglycerin, 0.4 mg.
   b) order a medical IV.
   c) perform a stat 12-lead electrocardiogram.
   d) order the appropriate bloodwork.
   e) order a gallbladder sonogram.

A 12-lead ECG has been performed (see Appendix Figure 2). Questioning conducted during performance of the ECG reveals that the patient has no known allergies, has had only one hospitalization other than childbirth for a hysterectomy 3 years ago, has no other chronic illnesses, and has no history of significant injury.

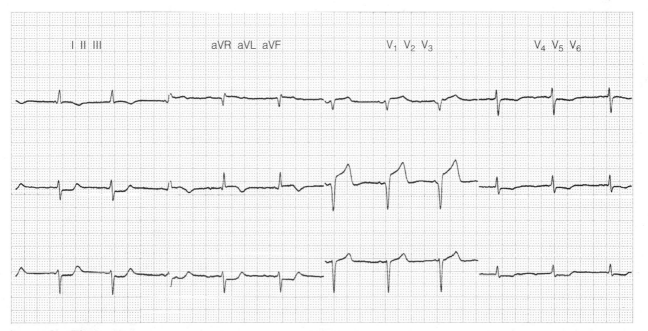

Appendix Figure 2

5. Upon completion of the ECG, you quickly note that the patient's electro-cardiogram shows
   a) a normal axis.
   b) right axis deviation.
   c) left axis deviation.
   d) an indeterminate axis.

6. On the basis of currently available information, you conclude that thrombolytic agents, if they were to be needed, would be
   a) absolutely contraindicated.
   b) relatively contraindicated.
   c) not contraindicated.

7. With regard to contraindications to aspirin, should it be necessary, you conclude that
   a) contraindications exist.
   b) no contraindications exist.

8. Upon further examination of the ECG, you conclude that it shows
   a) an acute inferior MI.
   b) an acute anterior MI.
   c) an inferior MI that may be old.
   d) an anterior MI that may be old.
   e) benign early repolarization changes.
   f) left bundle branch block simulating anterior MI.
   g) acute pericarditis.
   h) a normal ECG.
   i) nonspecific ST changes.

9. Your next procedural step should be to
   a) order sublingual nitroglycerin, 0.4 mg.
   b) order Maalox, 30 ml po.
   c) order a gallbladder sonogram.
   d) order a repeat ECG in 15 minutes.

The patient reports no relief from sublingual nitroglycerin, and a repeat ECG is unchanged from the first.

10. At this point, you conclude that
    a) sufficient evidence of AMI exists to initiate thrombolytic therapy, and you order the thrombolytic protocol.
    b) sufficient evidence of AMI exists to initiate thrombolytic therapy if blood pressure can be reduced below 180/110.
    c) evidence of AMI exists, but absolute contraindications prohibit thrombolytic therapy.
    d) evidence of AMI exists, but relative contraindications rule out thrombolytic therapy.
    e) insufficient evidence of AMI exists to initiate thrombolytic therapy. Further workup is necessary to establish a diagnosis.
    f) insufficient evidence of AMI exists to initiate thrombolytic therapy at present, but the index of suspicion is still high enough to warrant monitoring and repeat ECGs while a workup is proceeding.

ANSWERS AND CASE DISCUSSION

1.a   2.a   3.b   4.c   5.c   6.b   7.b   8.b   9.a   10.b

This middle-aged white female had significant risk factors in the form of obesity, hypertension, and diabetes, even though no family members were known to have had a myocardial infarction. Although the description of her pain, its radiation, and the way she related the pain to a fatty meal could suggest gallbladder disease, it is also entirely compatible with AMI. Nausea, vomiting, diaphoresis, and a mild sensation of shortness of breath could be common to both.

Important aspects of the physical examination included wet skin and an S4 gallop. Both findings are compatible with AMI, but wet skin also can be present in patients who are vomiting and in pain with acute cholecystitis, and an S4 gallop may be seen with hypertension alone. Nevertheless, the findings increase the index of suspicion for, and lend support to, a potential diagnosis of AMI.

Measures taken immediately to protect life are always the most important, so starting an IV would be your first order of priorities as the physician responsible for this patient. As usual, a stat 12-lead ECG should be performed prior to a therapeutic trial of nitroglycerin.

The ECG shows left axis deviation with an axis of about $-50°$, a small Q in lead I, and a small R wave in lead III. Therefore, criteria are present for left anterior hemiblock. ST segment elevation is present in the anterior wall in V_1 through V_3, with a slight upwardly convex ST elevation also seen in leads I and aVL. Reciprocal depression is present in the inferior and lateral walls. Q waves have formed in leads V_1 and V_2, and there is only a tiny R wave left in V_3. These findings indicate acute anterior wall myocardial infarction. A quick trial of nitroglycerin should be the next step to be certain that ST elevation is not on the basis of coronary artery spasm, although this is highly unlikely in the presence of developing Q waves.

Thrombolytic agents, on the basis of available information, are relatively contraindicated because of the patient's blood pressure in excess of 180/110, but they should be administered if treatment is successful in reducing blood pressure to 180/110 or below. This often can be accomplished simply with morphine and nitroglycerin. Additional beta-blockers also should be considered, since the patient remains hypertensive, with a heart rate in the 90s despite being on oral metoprolol. Aspirin is not contraindicated because there is no reported allergy to aspirin.

CASE NUMBER 3

You are functioning as a staff nurse in the cardiac care unit of a rural community hospital on the night shift. It is 2:35 AM. One of your assigned patients is Mr. Fitzgerald, a 54-year-old white male auto parts dealer who was admitted to the CCU at 7:00 PM the evening before with a chief complaint of 20 minutes of retrosternal pressure that came on as he was walking to his car through the parking lot after closing. He reported that he had experienced similar discomfort three or four times in the last several weeks with walking long distances, but that previous episodes had never been this severe or lasted as long as 20 minutes.

His pain had faded by the time of arrival in the emergency department, and an initial ECG and enzyme studies had been negative. Nonetheless, he had been admitted to the CCU by his family physician with a preliminary diagnosis of unstable angina. Your review of the admitting nursing notes had revealed that he is a one and a half pack a day smoker, and leads a sedentary life. He is not on medication and actually has not seen a physician in several years. His father had coronary artery bypass surgery at 70 years of age. He has no known allergies.

Mr. Fitzgerald has a keep-vein-open IV line of 5% dextrose and water and is connected to the ECG and noninvasive BP monitors. He is not on oxygen at present. His only current medication orders are for a nitroglycerin patch; phenergan, 12.5 mg IV q2h prn; and sublingual nitroglycerin, 0.4 mg prn. You are sitting at the central monitoring station doing chart work when you hear his call bell.

As you enter the room you note that he remains in normal sinus rhythm and that his monitor is displaying a blood pressure of 108/86. As you grasp his hand and ask what he needs, you note that his skin feels cool and diaphoretic. Mr. Fitzgerald stoically reports that his retrosternal pain of earlier this evening returned about 30 minutes ago but is now more severe. He appears uncomfortable and is moving almost constantly in the bed. Suddenly he sits up and emits a large amount of vomitus.

1. Your first action would be to
    a) administer 12.5 mg of phenergan IV.
    b) start oxygen.
    c) administer 0.4 mg of sublingual nitroglycerin.
    d) perform a 12-lead ECG.

2. Your second action would be to
    a) administer 12.5 mg of phenergan IV.
    b) start oxygen.
    c) administer 0.4 mg of sublingual nitroglycerin.
    d) perform a 12-lead ECG.

Your quick preliminary physical examination reveals diaphoretic skin, no jugular venous distention, and clear lungs. Vital signs are pulse, 78; respirations, 24; and BP, 108/86. A 12-lead ECG has been performed and is reproduced in Appendix Figure 3.

3. On the basis of currently available information, you conclude that thrombolytic agents, if they were to be needed, would be
    a) absolutely contraindicated.
    b) relatively contraindicated.
    c) not contraindicated.

4. With regard to contraindications to aspirin, should it be necessary, you conclude that
    a) contraindications exist.
    b) no contraindications exist.

5. Upon completion of the ECG, you quickly note that the patient's electrocardiogram shows
    a) a normal axis.
    b) right axis deviation.
    c) left axis deviation.
    d) an indeterminate axis.

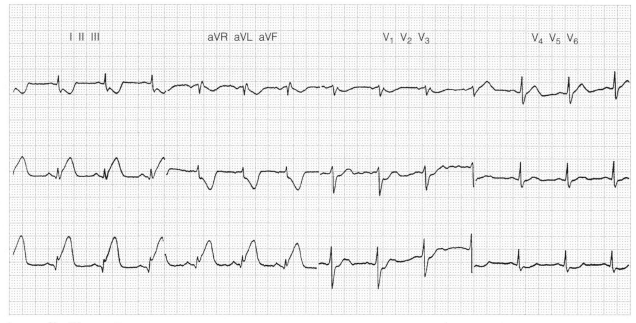

| I II III | aVR aVL aVF | $V_1 V_2 V_3$ | $V_4 V_5 V_6$ |

Appendix Figure 3

6. You place a call to the attending physician, report the events of the last 10 minutes, and report that it is your interpretation that the ECG shows
   a) an acute inferior MI.
   b) an acute anterior MI.
   c) an inferior MI that may be old.
   d) an anterior MI that may be old.
   e) benign early repolarization changes.
   f) left bundle branch block.
   g) right bundle branch block.
   h) acute pericarditis.
   i) nonspecific ST changes.
   j) a normal ECG.

7. When questioned by the physician, you further report that in your opinion
   a) sufficient evidence of AMI exists to recommend thrombolytic therapy.
   b) sufficient evidence of AMI exists to recommend thrombolytic therapy if a therapeutic trial of sublingual nitroglycerin does not resolve ST segment elevation.
   c) evidence of AMI exists, but absolute contraindications prohibit thrombolytic therapy.
   d) evidence of AMI exists, but relative contraindications rule out thrombolytic therapy.
   e) insufficient evidence of AMI exists to recommend thrombolytic therapy.

ANSWERS AND CASE DISCUSSION

1.b   2.d   3.c   4.b   5.a   6.a   7.b

This middle-aged white male was admitted with an unsubstantiated clinical diagnosis of unstable angina. He carried risk factors of smoking and a sedentary lifestyle. His father clearly had coronary artery disease, although not at a terribly young age. The history of his chest discomfort over the preceding several weeks is a fairly typical one for new onset of angina.

In the CCU he develops recurrence of retrosternal pain associated with nausea, vomiting, and diaphoresis, certainly a symptom complex compatible with AMI. The diaphoresis present on physical examination increases our index of suspicion for AMI.

The first appropriate step in managing this patient would be to start oxygen, an important step in protecting the patient that takes only seconds. The next step would be to perform a 12-lead ECG immediately. As discussed in previous cases, a therapeutic trial of nitroglycerin should be delayed until the ECG is performed, in order to avoid obscuring the diagnosis.

The ECG in this patient leaves little doubt about the cause of his symptoms. The axis is normal at about 90°, but there is dramatic ST elevation in leads II, III, and aVF, with reciprocal depression in leads I, aVL, and V_2 and V_3. Early pathologic Q wave formation also has begun in III and aVF. It is a classic ECG of acute inferior wall myocardial infarction.

There is nothing in the history to suggest contraindications to either thrombolytics or aspirin. The question arises whether or not to administer a therapeutic trial of nitroglycerin to someone who already has a nitroglycerin patch. In the absence of hypotension, most clinicians would still administer a dose of rapid-acting nitroglycerin. Thrombolytic therapy is clearly indicated in this patient if a subsequent therapeutic trial of nitroglycerin does not resolve the ST elevation.

CASE NUMBER 4

Today you are again assigned to an ALS unit in a large metropolitan area. It is 7:45 AM. Your unit is dispatched to an apartment building to investigate a person with chest pain and shortness of breath. In a fourth floor apartment you find 80-year-old Mr. Burgman wearing pajamas, sitting in his bedroom in a reclining chair. You immediately note that he appears very short of breath. Light from the overhead fixture is reflecting off his wet skin. As you approach his chair, you can hear respiratory wheezes even before you reach for your stethoscope. Multiple bottles of medicine are scattered on the nightstand beside him. Mr. Burgman relates to you that he has been short of breath and his chest has felt very tight since about 5 AM. He is also nauseated but has not yet vomited. He has broken out in a cold sweat in the last half hour.

With considerable effort, Mr. Burgman gasps that he has heart problems and has had three heart attacks, the last one a year ago. He has no known allergies. The medications on his nightstand include digoxin, 0.125 mg qd; furosemide, 40 mg bid; enalapril, 5 mg bid; sublingual nitroglycerin, 0.4 mg; and a transdermal nitroglycerin.

Your preliminary physical examination reveals an elderly white male who is in moderately severe respiratory distress and is able to speak only in short phrases because of dyspnea. Vital signs are a pulse of 92, respirations of 32, and a BP of 164/94. The skin is cool and damp. He is using his accessory muscles of inspiration. The neck veins are filled to the mandible. Basilar rales are present about a third of the way up the lung fields bilaterally, and there are diffuse expiratory wheezes. Heart sounds are distant and obscured by the wheezes and rales. The underlying rhythm is regular, but you hear occasional premature beats. There is +1 peripheral pitting edema at the ankles.

1. With regard to the history, you conclude that
    a) the history is compatible with AMI (acute myocardial infarction).
    b) the history is incompatible with AMI.

While you have been gathering a brief history and performing your examination, your partner has placed Mr. Burgman on oxygen by nonrebreather mask, placed him on a cardiac monitor and pulse oximeter, and started an IV of 5% dextrose and water. The monitor shows him to be in normal sinus rhythm with occasional unifocal premature ventricular contractions. His oxygen saturation is 88% on the nonrebreather mask.

2. Your next procedural step would be to
    a) administer nitroglycerin, 0.4 mg sublingually.
    b) administer furosemide, 80 mg IV.
    c) obtain a 12-lead electrocardiogram.
    d) administer lidocaine, 75 mg IV.
    e) administer a unit dose of nebulized albuterol sulfate.
    f) start another twin-catheter IV.
    g) administer aspirin, 325 mg.

3. Your next procedural step would be to
    a) administer nitroglycerin, 0.4 mg sublingually.
    b) administer furosemide, 80 mg IV.
    c) obtain a 12-lead electrocardiogram.
    d) administer lidocaine, 75 mg IV.
    e) administer a unit dose of nebulized albuterol sulfate.
    f) start another twin-catheter IV.
    g) administer aspirin, 325 mg.

While performing the foregoing procedures, you are able to elicit no further history that would contraindicate thrombolytic therapy. An ECG has been performed and is now available to you as it appears in Appendix Figure 4.

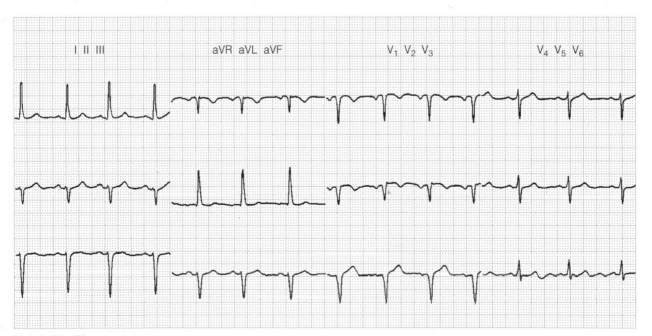

Appendix Figure 4

4. On the basis of currently available information you conclude that thrombolytic agents, if they were needed, would be
   a) absolutely contraindicated.
   b) relatively contraindicated.
   c) not contraindicated.

5. Upon completion of the ECG, you quickly note that the patient's electrocardiogram shows
   a) a normal axis.
   b) right axis deviation.
   c) left axis deviation
   d) an indeterminate axis.

6. Upon further examination of the ECG, you conclude that it shows
   a) an acute inferior MI.
   b) an acute anterior MI.
   c) an inferior MI that may be old.
   d) an anterior MI that may be old.
   e) benign early repolarization changes.
   f) left bundle branch block simulating anterior MI.
   g) acute pericarditis.
   h) a normal ECG.
   i) nonspecific ST changes.

7. Your partner has established contact with medical command. Your field assessment, as reported to the command physician, is that
   a) sufficient evidence of AMI exists to recommend thrombolytic therapy and to institute the prehospital thrombolytic protocol.
   b) evidence of AMI exists, but absolute contraindications prohibit thrombolytic therapy.
   c) evidence of AMI exists, but relative contraindications rule out thrombolytic therapy.
   d) insufficient evidence of AMI exists to recommend either thrombolytic therapy or implementation of the prehospital thrombolytic protocol.
   e) insufficient evidence of AMI exists to recommend thrombolytic therapy at present, but the index of suspicion is still high enough to warrant implementation of the prehospital thrombolytic protocol.

ANSWERS AND CASE DISCUSSION

1.a 2.b 3.c 4.c 5.c 6.d 7.e

Mr. Burgman is representative of a frequently encountered group of patients who can often be diagnostically challenging with regard to the presence or absence of acute myocardial infarction. He is an elderly patient with a long past medical history of cardiac disease, including his report of three previous heart attacks. His story of heart disease is corroborated by the medicines seen scattered on his nightstand. A quick glance at the patient upon entering the room is sufficient to tell that he is in trouble. He is in acute respiratory distress and is diaphoretic. He reports tightness in his chest as well as shortness of breath.

Usually at this early point we unconsciously begin to formulate a differential diagnosis in our minds and begin to ask ourselves questions. When Mr. Burgman says his chest is tight, does he mean that it is hard for him to take a breath because of the obvious bronchospasm, or does he mean that he has the constrictive feeling in his chest that people report with acute myocardial infarction? Is he short of breath and wheezing because he has chronic obstructive pulmonary disease (COPD) with respiratory failure, or because he is in pulmonary edema?

A brief physical examination confirms that he is, indeed, in acute pulmonary edema. The presence of jugular venous distention, peripheral edema, and rales at the bases, and his current array of medications that are aimed at congestive heart failure, help us feel confident that his repiratory distress is on the basis of pulmonary edema rather than COPD with bronchospasm. Now we face the question of whether Mr. Burgman's problem is acute pulmonary edema alone, or whether it is acute pulmonary edema precipitated by AMI. Clearly the history is potentially compatible with both.

Before we have the luxury of answering that question, we must care for Mr. Burgman's immediately life-threatening problem. So our first procedural step would be to administer furosemide, 80 mg IV, since we usually double the patient's oral dose when treating acute pulmonary edema. Nitroglycerin, of course, also can be beneficial in acute pulmonary edema by reducing preload and to a lesser extent afterload, but perhaps it would be best to wait until after an ECG has been performed to avoid the possibility of resolving ST segment elevation before we have had the opportunity to see the ECG. Albuterol can also be useful as an adjunct for the reflex bronchospasm associated with pulmonary edema, but it is not a first-line drug for pulmonary edema. Mr. Burgman does have premature ventricular contractions, but they are unifocal and are seen only occasionally, so indications are not yet present for lidocaine.

With an IV line established and oxygen and furosemide now on board, we can perform a quick ECG. We have not yet discovered any contraindications to thrombolytic therapy, and we know that Mr. Burgman's age is not a contraindication.

A glance at our ECG reveals that left axis deviation is present with an axis of perhaps −40 or −50 degrees. A small R is present in lead III and a small Q in lead I, so we are approaching criteria for left anterior hemiblock. We also note that the QRS duration approaches 0.10 sec in some leads, so there appears to be a mild intraventricular conduction delay. Most striking, however, are the Q waves we see in V_1 through V_3, indicating anterior wall infarction. The question then becomes, is the infarction old or new? There is slight ST elevation of less than 2 mm in V_2 and V_3, but we known that slight ST elevation often can persist in the anterior wall after large anterior infarctions. If we look for reciprocal depression, none is present on this tracing. We must conclude, therefore, that this tracing is most consistent with an old anterior MI. Furthermore, we also know that Mr. Burgman reports that he has had a heart attack in the past, a history compatible with the finding of an old MI on the ECG.

We are thus left with a history that is compatible with AMI but not compelling for AMI. In addition, we have a history of previous MI and an ECG that is more compatible with a remote infarction than with an acute infarction. Our assessment reported to medical command, therefore, should be that there is insufficient evidence of AMI to recommend thrombolytic therapy at the present, but since acute pulmonary edema is an occasional presenting symptom of AMI, prudence would dictate that we proceed with the prehospital protocol until subsequent evaluation in the emergency department (including a repeat ECG and, most importantly, comparison to an old ECG) could enhance our confidence that AMI was not present.

Although performing and assessing a field ECG takes only 3 to 4 minutes, additional measures to treat his pulmonary edema should take precedence over the ECG if this patient were to deteriorate or not improve after oxygen and furosemide. Such additional measures could include morphine sulfate, nitroglycerin, albuterol administration, or intubation.

CASE NUMBER 5

You are an independent primary health care provider working in a rural clinic in a western state. You are 70 miles from the nearest hospital, so your clinic also functions as the region's only emergency facility. You therefore have access to all ALS equipment and drugs, including thrombolytics. It is two o'clock in the afternoon.

Your receptionist has inserted a walk-in patient in your busy afternoon schedule because the patient is complaining of chest pain. You enter the room designated for emergencies and find a 54-year-old white female who appears anxious but in no immediate distress. Your assistant has placed her on oxygen and has connected her to the cardiac monitor. You quickly note that the patient is in normal sinus rhythm.

Mrs. Anderson is a cook in your town's only restaurant. You have been treating her with hydrochlorothiazide for mild hypertension for 3 years. She relates to you that she has had gradually increasing pain above her left breast and in her left shoulder and upper arm since approximately 10 AM today. She was unable to lift a frying pan with her left arm during the lunch rush today because of pain and weakness and had to use her right arm. There is no history of a previous similar pain. She denies nausea, vomiting, diaphoresis, or shortness of breath.

You glance at the patient's chart and note the vital signs that have been recorded by your assistant: pulse, 73; respirations, 18; blood pressure, 168/92. Mrs. Anderson is moderately obese. Her skin is warm and dry. There is no jugular venous distention. Her lungs are clear. Cardiac rhythm is regular without obvious gallops or murmurs. She is exquisitely tender to palpation over the head of her left biceps tendon. The abdomen is soft and nontender. There is no peripheral edema.

1. With regard to the pain, on the basis of currently available information you conclude that
    a) the history is adequate to be compatible with AMI (acute myocardial infarction).
    b) the history is not compatible with AMI.

2. With regard to the physical examination, you conclude that
    a) the physical examination lends support to the diagnosis of AMI.
    b) the physical examination neither confirms nor denies the possibility of AMI.

3. Your first procedural step would be to
    a) start an IV of 5% dextrose and water.
    b) administer nitroglycerin, 0.4 mg sublingually.
    c) perform a 12-lead electrocardiogram.

A review of Mrs. Anderson's chart while the chosen procedure is being performed reveals only the past medical history of hypertension and a hospitalization for a cystocele repair in 1984. Her parents are both still living. There is no history of bleeding, tumors, trauma, cerebrovascular accident, or recent surgery. She has no known allergies.

4. On the basis of currently available information you conclude that thrombolytic agents, if they were to be needed, would be
    a) absolutely contraindicated.
    b) relatively contraindicated.
    c) not contraindicated.

5. With regard to contraindications to aspirin, should it be necessary, you conclude that
    a) contraindications exist.
    b) no contraindications exist.

An ECG has been performed and is now available to you. It is reproduced in Appendix Figure 5A.

6. Upon completion of the ECG, you quickly note that the patient's electrocardiogram shows
    a) a normal axis.
    b) right axis deviation.
    c) left axis deviation.
    d) an indeterminate axis.

7. Upon further examination of the ECG, you conclude that it shows
    a) an acute inferior MI.
    b) an acute anterior MI.
    c) an inferior MI that may be old.
    d) an anterior MI that may be old.
    e) benign early repolarization changes.
    f) left bundle branch block simulating anterior MI.
    g) right bundle branch block.
    h) acute pericarditis.

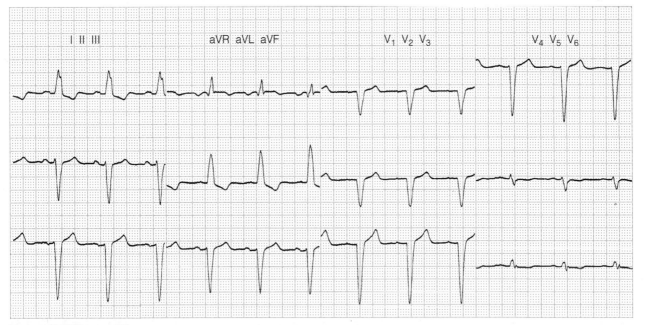

Appendix Figure 5A

  i) a normal ECG.
  j) nonspecific ST changes.

8. Your next procedural step would be to
  a) administer a therapeutic trial of nitroglycerin, 0.4 mg sublingually.
  b) administer morphine sulfate, 4 mg IV.
  c) compare the current ECG to an old one on the chart.

An ECG taken 2 years previously is shown in Appendix Figure 5B.

9. With regard to thrombolytic therapy, you conclude that
  a) sufficient evidence of AMI exists to initiate thrombolytic therapy and transport the patient by helicopter to the nearest hospital.
  b) sufficient evidence of AMI exists to initiate thrombolytic therapy, if a therapeutic trial of sublingual nitroglycerin does not resolve ST segment elevation.
  c) evidence of AMI exists, but absolute contraindications prohibit thrombolytic therapy.
  d) evidence of AMI exists, but relative contraindications rule out thrombolytic therapy.
  e) insufficient evidence of AMI exists to initiate thrombolytic therapy.

ANSWERS AND CASE DISCUSSION

1.b 2.b 3.c 4.c 5.b 6.c 7.f 8.c 9.e

Mrs. Anderson appeared in your clinic with a common presentation of chest pain. Her pain was located in the upper left anterior chest, left shoulder, and left upper arm. The most important historical finding is that the pain was clearly aggravated by the use of muscle groups in the same location as her pain. There is no history suggestive of unstable angina, since she never had a previous similar pain. Nausea, vomiting, diaphoresis, and shortness of breath were absent. This is not a history compatible with AMI but rather almost certainly represents chest wall pain coming from muscle inflammation or spasm.

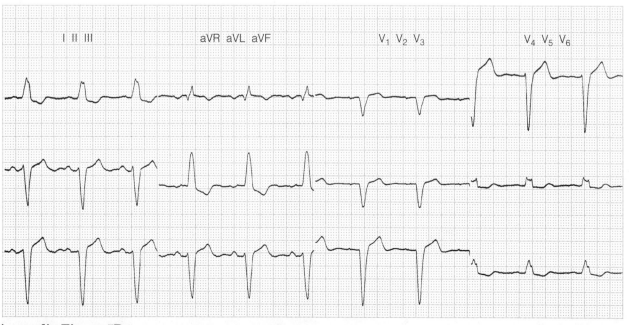

Appendix Figure 5B

The physical examination does nothing to heighten our index of suspicion for AMI but instead supports a diagnosis of biceps tendinitis because she is exquisitely tender over the head of the biceps tendon. It is common for muscle or tendon inflammation in the left shoulder to radiate into the pectoral muscles of the left chest wall and vice versa. Nevertheless, we know that AMI frequently presents without cardiovascular abnormalities on physical examination, so for the sake of thoroughness, we prudently perform a 12-lead electrocardiogram. Because both the history and physical examination so clearly lend support to a diagnostic category of musculoskeletal pain, it is not necessary to start an IV at this time.

You may have been initially disquieted to see Mrs. Anderson's ECG. She has an intraventricular conduction delay because the QRS is 0.12 second or greater, and it is of the left bundle branch block type. Her axis is about −70°. We know that all bets are off with regard to diagnosing AMI in the presence of left bundle branch block, so we are not very reassured by this electrocardiogram. We therefore look for an old ECG in her chart and find that she has had a left bundle branch block for at least 2 years. We note that her current ECG is unchanged from the one on file. Now we can breathe easier. There is no evidence of AMI, and the history and physical examination are clearly compatible with biceps tendinitis. A week of rest and anti-inflammatory medication and Mrs. Anderson will be back in the restaurant.

CASE NUMBER 6

You are a staff nurse in a community hospital emergency department. It is a busy Friday night at 9:30 PM. The sole physician on duty is suturing an extensive dog bite wound when the triage nurse brings in a 62-year-old black male with chest pain and turns the patient over to you. Mr. Federick transfers from the wheelchair to the stretcher. He appears to be in pain. He relates to you that he has had retrosternal chest pain, radiating into both upper arms, for 30 minutes. As you are placing him on oxygen by nasal cannula at 6 liters and connecting him to the monitoring equipment, you note that his skin appears warm and dry and that he does not appear to be in respiratory distress. The monitor shows normal sinus rhythm at a rate of 80. The noninvasive blood pressure module reads 134/82. His oxygen saturation is 98% on oxygen. You quickly listen to his lungs, and they are clear. You can see no jugular venous distention. His heart rhythm is regular, and you can hear no gross murmurs or gallops. His abdomen is soft and nontender. There is no peripheral edema.

You prepare to start an IV line. Further questioning during this task reveals that he has been having chest discomfort about once a week for about 2 years. The discomfort usually comes with exercise, such as taking out the trash, and goes away within 2 to 3 minutes when he takes a nitroglycerin tablet or sits and rests for 5 minutes. He is maintained on diltiazem, 60 mg tid, and sustained release propranolol, 80 mg bid. Tonight's pain came on at rest while he was watching TV after dinner, and it has been unrelieved by one sublingual nitroglycerin. He has never had pain this long. He has had no nausea and vomiting, diaphoresis, or shortness of breath. He denies allergies to medications.

1. With regard to the pain, on the basis of currently available information you conclude that
    a) the history is adequate to be compatible with AMI.
    b) the history is not compatible with AMI.

2. With regard to the physical examination, you conclude that
    a) the physical examination lends support to the diagnosis of AMI.

b) the physical examination neither confirms nor denies the possibility of AMI.

3. You have completed starting the IV and have drawn blood in the process. Your next step is to
   a) administer nitroglycerin, 0.4 mg sublingually.
   b) administer aspirin, 325 mg PO.
   c) perform a stat 12 lead-electrocardiogram.
   d) start two more IV lines.
   e) order a stat portable chest film.

Further questioning reveals no historical contraindications to thrombolytic therapy. A 12-lead ECG has been performed and is reproduced in Appendix Figure 6.

4. Upon completion of the ECG, you quickly note that the patient's electrocardiogram shows
   a) a normal axis.
   b) right axis deviation.
   c) left axis deviation.
   d) an indeterminate axis.

5. Upon further examination of the ECG, you conclude that it shows
   a) an acute inferior MI.
   b) an acute anterior MI.
   c) an inferior MI that may be old.
   d) an anterior MI that may be old.
   e) ST depression compatible with ischemia.
   f) left bundle branch block simulating anterior MI.
   g) right bundle branch block.
   h) acute pericarditis.
   i) a normal ECG.
   j) nonspecific ST changes.

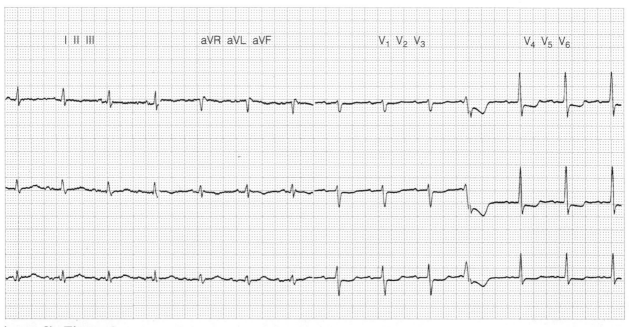

Appendix Figure 6

6. After presenting a report to the physician who is suturing the dog bite wound, and showing him the ECG, he is most likely to order you to
   a) begin the thrombolytic protocol.
   b) start a nitroglycerin drip.
   c) administer aspirin, 325 mg PO.
   d) complete the cardiac workup with a chest film.
   e) administer morphine sulfate, 4 mg IV.

ANSWERS AND CASE DISCUSSION

1.a   2.b   3.c   4.a   5.e   6.b

This middle-aged black male presents with a history of stable angina under current treatment with calcium channel blockers, beta-blockers, and prn nitroglycerin. His pain usually comes with exertion, but today it came at rest and has continued for 30 minutes through to the time of admission. Although he has had no nausea, vomiting, diaphoresis, or shortness of breath, his pain almost certainly represents heart pain, and his symptoms are certainly compatible with AMI. We are not surprised that his physical examination is unrevealing, and we conclude that it neither confirms nor denies the possibility of AMI.

We have taken measures to protect our patient from a sudden adverse event right up front with oxygen, monitoring, and starting an IV. Before we start any other form of therapy or do any other investigative test, our first order of business is now to obtain an ECG as quickly as possible. Up to this point we have discovered no contraindications to thrombolytic therapy should the ECG confirm AMI.

The ECG does not, however, show any ST elevation. Rather there is ST depression of 2 mm or greater in leads V_4 and V_5. The ST segments are fairly straight and form a fairly acute angle with the T wave. This tracing is compatible with severe ischemia, but does not yet show AMI. At this point we have a classic case of unstable angina. In this context, our physician is most likely to order a nitroglycerin drip as the first and most important therapeutic step, now that the diagnosis seems confirmed. Other diagnostic and therapeutic measures may follow his first-line intervention.

CASE NUMBER 7

It is 11:30 AM on Sunday morning. Your ALS unit is dispatched to a local church for a person with chest pain. As you pull into the church parking lot, a man is frantically waving toward the open church door. In the church vestibule a middle-aged white man is lying motionless, supine on the floor, his head in a pool of vomitus. A woman is kneeling over him, screaming hysterically. A teenager is giving the man closed chest massage, but he is not being ventilated. Your partner is already unpacking the defibrillator as you reach for a pulse, but none is present. As you rip open the man's shirt you ask a bystander how long ago he collapsed and he answers 1 minute, maybe 2, before you arrived. The stricken man takes a sudden agonal gasp but is otherwise not breathing.

1. Your first action will be to
   a) start an IV.
   b) begin bag-valve-mask ventilation.
   c) connect the patient to a monitor and defibrillate if ventricular fibrillation is present.
   d) intubate.

As the monitor baseline settles down, you immediately recognize a pattern of coarse ventricular fibrillation. A shock at 200 joules is ineffective. After a second shock at 300 joules, there is a brief moment of asystole, followed by return of a sinus bradycardia that slowly increases in rate to a sinus tachycardia. You are able to feel a brisk carotid pulse with each QRS.

2. Your second action will be to
    a) clear the airway and ventilate with bag-valve-mask while your partner assembles intubation gear
    b) start an IV.
    c) administer epinephrine, 1 mg IV.
    d) administer lidocaine, 75 mg IV.

Your patient begins to breathe spontaneously very shortly after defibrillation and is now beginning to stir. You decide not to intubate. As your partner starts the IV, you learn from your patient's wife that he had 15 minutes of severe chest pain and broke out in a sweat before they got out of a pew and called 911. He vomited and then collapsed just before you arrived. His total period of arrest and CPR was probably under 4 minutes. His wife is not aware of any allergies. He is not on any medications.

Lidocaine, 75 mg IV, is now on board, and a drip is running at 2 mg per minute. Mr. Seymour, as you now know his name to be, is moaning. His blood pressure is 132/78. His lungs are clear, and he is moving air well. He is being loaded into the ambulance.

3. Your next action will be to
    a) administer nitroglycerin spray under the tongue.
    b) perform a 12-lead ECG.
    c) administer aspirin, 325 mg.
    d) administer morphine sulfate, 4 mg IV.

A 12-lead ECG is now available to you and is pictured in Appendix Figure 7. Mr. Seymour is now alert enough to answer most questions. You have discovered nothing in his history that contraindicates thrombolytics.

4. You quickly note that the patient's electrocardiogram shows
    a) a normal axis.
    b) right axis deviation.
    c) left axis deviation.
    d) an indeterminate axis.

5. Upon further examination of the ECG, you conclude that it shows
    a) an acute inferior MI.
    b) an acute anterior MI.
    c) an inferior MI that may be old.
    d) an anterior MI that may be old.
    e) ST depression compatible with ischemia.
    f) left bundle branch block simulating anterior MI.
    g) right bundle branch block.
    h) acute pericarditis.
    i) a normal ECG.
    j) nonspecific ST changes.

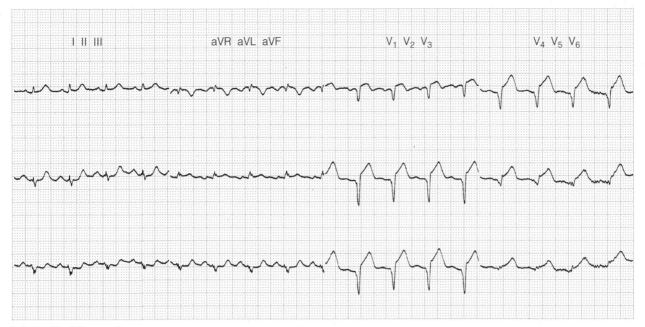

Appendix Figure 7

6. By this time you have concluded that thrombolytic therapy is
   a) contraindicated.
   b) not contraindicated.

7. Radio contact has been established with medical command. Your field assessment as reported to the command physician is that
   a) sufficient evidence of AMI exists to recommend thrombolytic therapy.
   b) evidence of AMI exists, but absolute contraindications prohibit thrombolytic therapy.
   c) evidence of AMI exists, but relative contraindications rule out thrombolytic therapy.
   d) insufficient evidence of AMI exists to recommend either thrombolytic therapy or implementation of the prehospital thrombolytic protocol.
   e) insufficient evidence of AMI exists to recommend thrombolytic therapy at present, but the index of suspicion is still high enough to warrant inplementation of the prehospital thrombolytic protocol.

ANSWERS AND CASE DISCUSSION

1.c   2.a   3.b   4.c   5.b   6.b   7.a

Up to 40% of cases of acute myocardial infarction present to the Emergency Medical Services system as sudden death. This patient had a down time of only 1 or 2 minutes prior to ALS arrival. Upon confirmation of absent pulse and respiration, the first priority is to rapidly determine rhythm and administer DC countershock if the patient is determined to be in ventricular fibrillation.

The second priority in this case was to clear the airway, quickly ventilate with bag-valve-mask, and prepare to intubate. When patients have a short period of arrest and are rapidly defibrillated with return of good cardiac output, intubation often is not necessary if adequate spontaneous respirations quickly resume. Such was the case with this patient. Starting an IV line and administering lidocaine are certainly appropriate measures in a patient who has just experienced ventricular fibrillation, but they are secondary to adequate ventilation. Epinephrine was not indicated.

Mr. Seymour's history is a classic one for AMI complicated by early ventricular fibrillation. By now you are familiar with the concept that performance of the 12-lead ECG should be accomplished prior to administering nitroglycerin. Aspirin is not indicated until the decision has been made to institute the prehospital thrombolytic protocol, which requires the completion of a 12-lead ECG. Morphine is usually not administered until nitroglycerin has failed to provide pain relief.

Mr. Seymour's ECG shows an axis of about $-15°$, so left axis deviation is present. Sinus tachycardia is present with a rate of slightly over 100. Prominent ST elevation is present in the anterior wall across the entire precordium, with reciprocal depression in the inferior wall indicating extensive anterior wall infarction. Q waves have already formed in V_1 through V_5.

No contraindications to thrombolytic therapy have been elicited, and although CPR over 10 minutes is a relative contraindication, Mr. Seymour's period of resuscitation was no more than 4 minutes. Thrombolytic therapy is indicated in this patient.

CASE NUMBER 8

It is 6:15 PM. You are starving. You and your ALS partner have just made your way through the cafeteria line and are sitting down to roast beef and lemon meringue pie when the tones go off. You are dispatched to a local residence for aid to a person with chest pain. Upon arrival, you recognize a familiar face. Sixty-four-year-old Mr. Saunders is well known to you, having a long history of coronary artery disease and having been transported to the hospital with chest pain three or four times in the last year and a half. His wife mentions to you that he was just discharged from the hospital 2 weeks ago after another heart attack.

Mr. Saunders reports to you that he is having retrosternal heaviness similar to that which he has had in the past when he had heart attacks. You quickly note as you are placing him on oxygen that his skin is warm and dry, and that he does not appear dyspneic. As your partner connects him to the cardiac monitor, Mr. Saunders relates that he has had the pain about 15 minutes, but that he has no nausea, vomiting, or shortness of breath with the pain.

1. Your first action will be to
    a) start an IV line.
    b) administer sublingual nitroglycerin, 0.4 mg.
    c) perform a 12-lead electrocardiogram.

2. Your second action will be to
    a) start an IV line.
    b) administer sublingual nitroglycerin, 0.4 mg.
    c) perform a 12-lead electrocardiogram.

Questioning during the foregoing procedures reveals that Mr. Saunders has had several heart attacks and a cardiac catheterization in the past and was hospitalized for a bleeding ulcer about one year ago. He had at least one hospitalization for congestive heart failure. He is allergic to procainamide, but no other drugs. He is currently maintained on a nitroglycerin patch; furosemide, 40 mg bid; captopril, 25 mg bid; digoxin, 0.125 mg every other day; and one aspirin daily. When asked specifically about "clot-busting drugs," he thinks he was given one with his last heart attack 3 weeks ago, but he is not sure of the name of the drug.

Your brief physical examination has revealed a pulse of 96, respirations of 18, and a blood pressure of 108/68. Mr. Saunders has no jugular venous distention, his lungs are clear, you cannot hear a cardiac gallop (although there seems to be a systolic murmur present), and there is no peripheral edema.

3. By now you have concluded that thrombolytic therapy, should it be a therapeutic consideration, would be
   a) contraindicated.
   b) relatively contraindicated.
   c) not contraindicated.

A 12-lead electrocardiogram has now been performed and is reproduced in Appendix Figure 8.

4. You quickly note that the ECG shows an axis of approximately
   a) −100°
   b) −60°
   c) 0°
   d) 60°
   e) 90°

5. Upon further examination of the ECG, you conclude that it shows (may select more than one answer)
   a) inferior MI that may be acute.
   b) anterior MI that may be acute.
   c) inferior MI that may be old.
   d) anterior MI that may be old.
   e) ST depression compatible with ischemia.
   f) left bundle branch block simulating anterior MI.
   g) right bundle branch block.

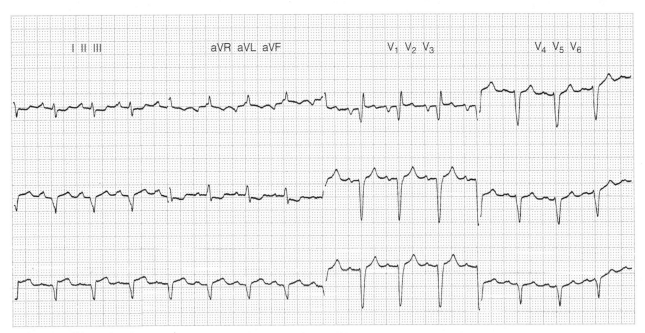

Appendix Figure 8

h) acute pericarditis.
i) a normal ECG.
j) nonspecific ST changes.

6. Radio contact has been established with medical command. Your field assessment, as reported to the command physician, is that
   a) sufficient evidence of AMI exists to recommend thrombolytic therapy.
   b) evidence of AMI exists, but absolute contraindications prohibit thrombolytic therapy.
   c) evidence of AMI exists, but relative contraindications rule out thrombolytic therapy.
   d) insufficient evidence of AMI exists to recommend either thrombolytic therapy or implementation of the prehospital thrombolytic protocol.
   e) insufficient evidence of AMI exists to recommend thrombolytic therapy at present, but the index of suspicion is still high enough to warrant implementation of the prehospital thrombolytic protocol.

7. The medical command physician is now likely to recommend that you administer
   a) aspirin, 325 mg, chewed.
   b) nitroglycerin, 0.4 mg, sublingually.
   c) morphine, 4 mg IV.
   d) lidocaine, 75 mg IV.

ANSWERS AND CASE DISCUSSION

1.a   2.c   3.c   4.a   5.a,d,e,g   6.e   7.b

Mr. Saunders is a very likely candidate for AMI. He has a history of several myocardial infarctions in the past, including one 3 weeks ago, as well as a history of congestive heart failure. His description of the pain that he is encountering this evening is that it feels about the same as the pain of his previous heart attacks. Clearly there is adequate history to have a very high index of suspicion for AMI.

You have a good partner who has already connected Mr. Saunders to the cardiac monitor while you were placing him on oxygen, and the last remaining immediate step to protect your patient would be to start an IV. Now you can perform a quick 12-lead ECG before nitroglycerin is administered.

By the end of your brief history and physical examination, you should have concluded that thrombolytic therapy was not contraindicated. Mr. Saunders does have a history of a bleeding ulcer, but it was about a year ago and does not contraindicate thrombolytic therapy. Indeed, he apparently had thrombolytic therapy with his last heart attack 3 weeks ago. Should you decide that thrombolytic therapy is indicated, you will need to check his old chart to see which thrombolytic agent was administered 3 weeks ago. If it was streptokinase, you would need to use another thrombolytic agent on this occasion because of the possible development of streptokinase antibodies.

Mr. Saunders' ECG shows extreme left axis deviation. Lead aVR is upright, and lead I is almost equally biphasic, so we place the axis at about $-100°$. Mr. Saunders' 12-lead ECG is very interesting and presents some real dilemmas. First, we note that the QRS duration is 0.12 sec or greater, and that there is a very prominent R prime deflection in lead V_1. This means that Mr. Saunders has a right bundle branch block. There is no R wave, however, in leads V_1 and V_2, and only the smallest of R waves in V_3 because Mr. Saunders has pathologic

Q waves indicative of an anterior wall infarction. However, there is no acute anterior wall ST elevation and no reciprocal depression in the inferior wall. Indeed, the inferior wall shows Q waves and ST elevation in leads II, III, and aVF. There is also some reciprocal depression in leads I and aVL, although there is none in the precordial leads. We therefore come to a tentative conclusion that the anterior wall infarction is probably old, but that the inferior wall infarction could be new because of the presence of inferior wall ST elevation and reciprocal depression in I and aVL.

Nevertheless, we also know that Mr. Saunders apparently just suffered a myocardial infarction 3 weeks ago, and it is possible that the ST elevation in the inferior wall could be from a recent inferior wall infarction that has not yet undergone resolution. Thus, both the anterior and inferior infarctions could be old. In that case, his current chest pain could represent unstable angina. Clearly, we are going to need to see an old tracing from his recent hospitalization before we can confidently tell whether the inferior wall infarction is new, or was suffered 3 weeks ago.

Since both the anterior and inferior wall infarctions may be old, we cannot currently recommend institution of thrombolytic therapy but can only recommend that the index of suspicion is still high enough to warrant proceeding to implement the prehospital thrombolytic protocol. Final decisions will have to await comparison of our field ECG with Mr. Saunders' old ECG in the emergency department.

Since Mr. Saunders is already taking an aspirin daily, our medical commander is likely to order sublingual nitroglycerin, now that we have obtained a 12-lead ECG.

So what was the outcome of this case? It was unstable angina. Mr. Saunders' field ECG, upon comparison with old tracings in the emergency department, was essentially unchanged from his last tracing 2 weeks prior when he was discharged from the hospital following an acute inferior wall myocardial infarction. A very challenging case! If you got all seven questions right in this case, you get a star.

CASE NUMBER 9

Despite the pressures of too many patients being jammed into every day's schedule, commuting 20 minutes to and from the hospital, and the necessity of taking calls every other night, rural family practice has always been your first love. This evening is no exception, with a waiting room full of coughing kids, pregnant young mothers, and the usual assortment of diabetics and hypertensives. You enter Examining Room 3 to see Ray Stoneham, a cheerful 68-year-old dairy farmer with a ruddy complexion, and a concerned wife who talked your receptionist into sticking him into tonight's packed schedule.

His wife pre-empts your attempt to take a history by announcing that Ray has had indigestion for 3 days, has been taking Tums by the bucketload, and just picks at his food. She is sure that he has an ulcer.

Ray seems content with his wife running this show and makes no effort to offer further clarification. The office chart in your hand is thin. Ray normally comes in only when coerced by his wife. He has never been in a hospital, has no chronic illnesses or allergies, and is on no medications. But tonight, his wife says, he himself suggested coming to the doctor's office. Gradually you are able to coax more information out of Ray, and you learn that his indigestion is high in the retrosternal area, has been constant for almost 3 days, and seems worse when he is carrying feed to the calves. He vomited once the first night of the indigestion and was sweaty most of the night. Tums have not seemed to relieve the indigestion.

During your questioning, you are working your way through a brief physical examination. You note that Ray's skin is warm and dry. There is no jugular venous distention. His lungs are clear. His cardiac rhythm is regular in the 80s with an occasional premature beat. There are no murmurs or gallops. His abdomen is soft and nontender. You are unable to reproduce his discomfort with palpation in the epigastrium. You note on the chart that his blood pressure is 148/92.

1. Your next step would be to
   a) call an ambulance.
   b) schedule an upper GI series.
   c) schedule a gallbladder sonogram.
   d) perform a stat electrocardiogram
   e) order screening chemistry and enzyme studies.
   f) start O_2 and an IV line, and connect Ray to your office monitor/defibrillator.

2. Your second step would be to
   a) call an ambulance.
   b) schedule an upper GI series.
   c) schedule a gallbladder sonogram.
   d) perform a stat electrocardiogram.
   e) order screening chemistry and enzyme studies.
   f) start O_2 and an IV line, and connect Ray to your office monitor/defibrillator.

An ECG has been performed and is now available (see Appendix Figure 9). There is no old tracing on file for comparison.

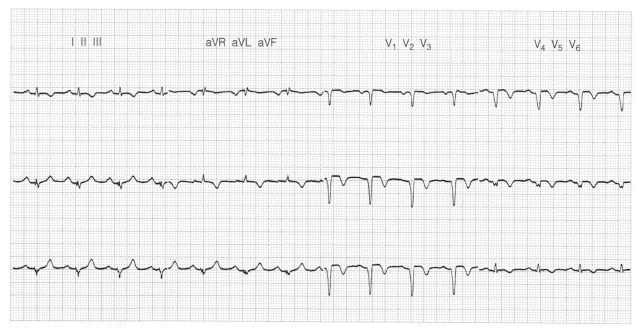

Appendix Figure 9

3. By now you have concluded that thrombolytic therapy, should it be a therapeutic consideration, would be
    a) contraindicated.
    b) relatively contraindicated.
    c) not contraindicated.

4. You quickly note that Mr. Stoneham's tracing shows
    a) left anterior hemiblock.
    b) left posterior hemiblock.
    c) nonspecific intraventricular conduction delay.
    d) right bundle branch block.
    e) left bundle branch block.
    f) normal QRS duration and axis.

5. In addition, Mr. Stoneham's tracing shows
    a) an evolving acute inferior MI.
    b) an evolving acute anterior MI.
    c) an inferior MI that may be old.
    d) an anterior MI that may be old.
    e) ST depression compatible with ischemia.
    f) left bundle branch block simulating anterior MI.
    g) right bundle branch block.
    h) acute pericarditis.
    i) a normal ECG.
    j) nonspecific ST changes.

6. By this time, you have concluded that Mr. Stoneham
    a) is a candidate for thrombolytic therapy.
    b) is not a candidate for thrombolytic therapy.

7. Your next step would be to
    a) call an ambulance.
    b) schedule an upper GI series.
    c) schedule a gallbladder sonogram.
    d) order screening chemistry and enzyme studies.
    e) start O$_2$ and an IV line, and connect Ray to your office monitor/defibrillator.

ANSWERS AND CASE DISCUSSION

1.f 2.d 3.c 4.a 5.b 6.b 7.a

Ray Stoneham is typical of a group of stoic patients who endure symptoms of cardiac disease and convince themselves that their symptoms represent something less serious. The first hint that this is not a GI problem comes when Ray relates that his "indigestion" is in the high retrosternal area. Aggravation of the pain with exercise sets off further alarm bells. Vomiting and diaphoresis the first night of the pain complete the transition to a focus on a possible cardiac etiology. Ray's symptoms, indeed, are sufficiently worrisome to warrant hospitalization regardless of our findings on physical examination or laboratory investigation.

The physical examination is not particularly helpful. The only positive finding is an occasional premature beat, which, taken alone, does not significantly heighten our index of suspicion for AMI. The absence of tenderness in the epigastrium does help heighten our suspicion that this illness is not gastrointestinal in etiology.

On the basis of the history alone, which is highly suspicious for AMI, our initial step would be to start O_2, connect Ray to a monitor/defibrillator, and start an IV line, if all were available in the office, to protect Ray from an adverse event like ventricular fibrillation. Our next step would be to perform a stat electrocardiogram.

Nothing in Ray's history suggests a contraindication to thrombolytics.

Ray's electrocardiogram is illuminating. Left axis deviation of approximately $-45°$, and a small Q in lead I and a very small R in lead III meet criteria for left anterior hemiblock. Most disturbing, however, are the Q waves in V_1 through V_3, with deep T wave inversion characteristic of an anterior wall myocardial infarction in evolution. The question arises: how old is this infarction? T wave inversion takes at least hours to days to evolve, so the ECG would suggest that it is probably at least more than several hours old.

Often, however, the most accurate way to judge the age of an evolving infarction is on the basis of the patient's history. Ray tells us that his pain has been constant for nearly 3 days, and that on the first night of the pain he had diaphoresis and vomiting. Clinically, then, the infarction commenced 3 days ago. Too late for thrombolytic therapy, but still early enough that he remains at some risk and should be hospitalized. Our final step would be to call 911 for an ambulance trip to the hospital with ALS services.

CASE NUMBER 10

When Robert Freuhauf was admitted to the coronary care unit, you learned during your nursing evaluation that he was unfortunate enough to have had a myocardial infarction 7 years previously at the age of 33. Robert had had a cardiac catheterization shortly thereafter, the results of which are unclear to you. He can only remember that they told him he had a "tear" in a vessel wall. After 7 years free of chest pain or other symptoms, Robert had been readmitted 2 weeks ago with a several-week history of exertional chest discomfort relieved by rest, and then finally an episode of pain at rest leading to admission. After several days in the CCU, Robert had had a treadmill stress test, which was negative, and he was discharged on aspirin and diltiazem.

Late this afternoon Robert again experienced an hour of severe retrosternal chest discomfort that began to ease at about the time of admission to the emergency department. Robert's emergency department ECG at 5:37 PM is seen in Appendix Figure 10A. It is unchanged from that of his previous admission.

1. Robert's emergency department ECG at 5:37 PM shows
   a) left anterior hemiblock.
   b) left posterior hemiblock.
   c) nonspecific intraventricular conduction delay.
   d) right bundle branch block.
   e) left bundle branch block.
   f) normal QRS duration and axis.

2. In addition, Robert's 5:37 PM tracing shows
   a) an acute inferior MI.
   b) an acute anterior MI.
   c) an inferior MI that may be old.
   d) an anterior MI that may be old.
   e) ST depression compatible with ischemia.

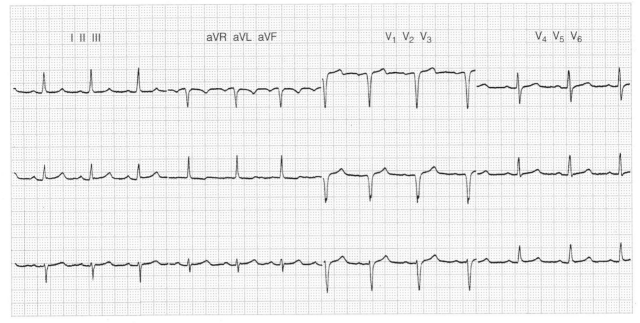

I II III   aVR aVL aVF   V₁ V₂ V₃   V₄ V₅ V₆

Appendix Figure 10A

f) left bundle branch block simulating anterior MI.
g) right bundle branch block.
h) acute pericarditis.
i) normal morphology.
j) nonspecific ST changes.

Robert has been pain-free since admission to the CCU 45 minutes ago. He is on oxygen at 2 liters by nasal cannula, has a keep-vein-open IV of 5% dextrose and water, and has a nitroglycerin drip running at 10 μg/min. He received 50 mg of metoprolol by mouth at 6:15 PM. His physician has written prn orders for morphine and an antacid. At approximately 6:30 PM he rings his call bell, and when you enter the room he tells you that the pain has returned. He rates the pain as an 8 on a scale of 10.

3. Your first step would be to
    a) increase the rate of the nitroglycerin drip.
    b) take vital signs and do a brief pertinent physical examination.
    c) administer morphine sulfate, 4 mg IV.
    d) perform a repeat 12-lead electrocardiogram.
    e) administer Maalox, 30 ml po.

4. Your second step would be to
    a) increase the rate of the nitroglycerin drip.
    b) take vital signs and do a brief pertinent physical examination.
    c) administer morphine sulfate, 4 mg IV.
    d) perform a repeat 12-lead electrocardiogram.
    e) administer Maalox, 30 ml po.

Robert's current vital signs are a pulse of 103, BP of 158/92, and respirations of 20. His skin is cool and slightly diaphoretic. There is no jugular venous distention. His lungs are clear, and there is no suggestion of a new murmur or gallop rhythm. A 12-lead electrocardiogram taken at 6:38 PM is reproduced in Appendix Figure 10B.

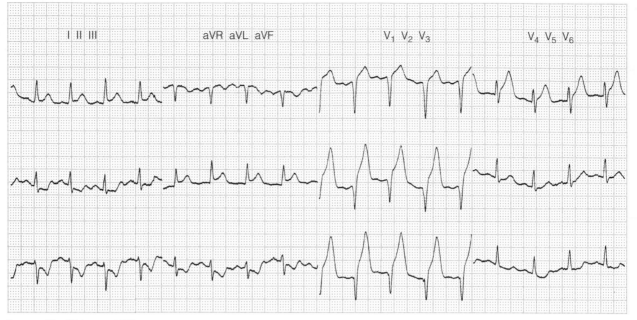

Appendix Figure 10B

5. Robert's 6:38 PM tracing shows
    a) an acute inferior MI.
    b) an acute anterior MI.
    c) an inferior MI that may be old.
    d) an anterior MI that may be old.
    e) ST depression compatible with ischemia.
    f) left bundle branch block simulating anterior MI.
    g) right bundle branch block.
    h) acute pericarditis.
    i) normal morphology.
    j) nonspecific ST changes.

6. Your next step would be to
    a) increase the rate of the nitroglycerin drip.
    b) take vital signs and do a brief pertinent physical examination.
    c) administer morphine sulfate, 4 mg IV.
    d) question the patient regarding thrombolytic contraindications and prepare for possible thrombolytic therapy.
    e) administer Maalox, 30 ml po.
    f) administer aspirin, 325 mg po.

Robert has received no relief of pain from the measures taken so far. You have been unable to contact Robert's physician by either pager or telephone. You have left him connected to the 12-lead ECG machine, and you note that there is no change from the previous 6:38 PM tracing.

7. Your next step would be to
    a) increase the rate of the nitroglycerin drip.
    b) take vital signs and do a brief pertinent physical examination.
    c) administer morphine sulfate, 4 mg IV.
    d) question the patient regarding thrombolytic contraindications and prepare for possible thrombolytic therapy.
    e) administer Maalox, 30 ml po.
    f) administer aspirin, 325 mg po.

ANSWERS AND
CASE DISCUSSION

1.f   2.d   3.b   4.d   5.b   6.a   7.d

This case illustrates the importance of maintaining a high index of suspicion and performing repeat ECGs in patients whose symptoms change. Robert is young and had a recent admission with a negative workup. In addition, although his emergency department ECG shows Q waves consistent with an old anterior MI, it is unchanged from that of his previous admission. It is easy to be lulled into a false sense of security by this history of a negative workup and continued negative ECGs without acute changes.

But once again, 45 minutes after admission, Robert experiences a return of his chest pain. As always, when a patient's condition changes, we need to check the patient. So the first step would be taking his vital signs and at least observing skin color and temperature, checking for jugular venous distention, and at least listening to his heart and lungs.

It would be tempting at this point to increase the nitroglycerin drip in an effort to relieve Robert's pain, but as we have learned in earlier cases, it is better quickly to perform a 12-lead ECG first in order not to miss a diagnosis.

The 12-lead ECG performed at 6:38 PM leaves no doubt of the etiology of Robert's pain. Dramatic ST elevation is present in the anterior wall, with reciprocal depression. It is now time to turn up the nitroglycerin drip to see whether higher doses relieve the pain and ST elevation.

You have prudently left Robert connected to the 12-lead machine (or, if you have ST segment monitoring in your CCU, you may have continuously monitored his ST segments). In the absence of relief, it is time to begin questioning the patient with regard to contraindications to thrombolytic therapy and prepare for thrombolytic therapy in anticipation of it being ordered. Morphine and aspirin administration could follow closely.

You may be interested to hear that in the real-life case, Robert's ST segment elevation and pain resolved within about 10 minutes of increasing the nitroglycerin drip. He was flown to a tertiary center where he underwent emergency cardiac catheterization. Immediately thereafter he was taken to the operating room where he underwent an uncomplicated triple coronary artery bypass.

Appendix 2

▦ Answers to Practice Tracings

CHAPTER 5

Figure 5–5: −5°
Figure 5–6: Slightly greater than 90°
Figure 5–7: 140°
Figure 5–8: −20°

CHAPTER 6

Figure 6–8: Left posterior hemiblock; axis 115°
Figure 6–9: Left anterior hemiblock; axis −45°
Figure 6–10: Left posterior hemiblock; axis 175°
Figure 6–11: Left anterior hemiblock; axis −70°

CHAPTER 7

Figure 7–18: Complete left bundle branch block; axis −20°
Figure 7–19: Incomplete left bundle branch block; axis −7°
Figure 7–20: Complete right bundle branch block and left anterior hemiblock; axis −55°
Figure 7–21: Incomplete right bundle branch block; axis 25°

CHAPTER 8

Figure 8–6: Left ventricular hypertrophy by voltage criteria and a typical strain pattern; axis 57°
Figure 8–7: Right ventricular hypertrophy with an R to S ratio in lead V_1 of greater than 1.0, right axis deviation, normal QRS duration, and a strain pattern in the limb leads with the tallest QRS; axis 100°

CHAPTER 9

Figure 9–17: Acute anterior wall infarction showing ST elevation in leads V_1 through V_5 and in aVL, with reciprocal depression in leads II, III, and aVF; axis approximately 60°.
Figure 9–18: Acute inferolateral wall infarction showing ST elevation in leads II, III, and aVF, and in V_5 and V_6. Reciprocal depression is present in leads V_1 through V_3 and in aVL. Early Q waves are present in leads III and aVF; axis is approximately 15°.
Figure 9–19: Acute inferior wall infarction showing ST elevation in leads II, III, and aVF, with reciprocal depression in leads I and aVL. Pathologic Q wave formation is incomplete. Axis is approximately 90°.
Figure 9–20: Extensive acute anterior wall infarction showing ST elevation in leads V_1 through V_6 and in aVL. Pathologic Q waves are present in leads V_1 through V_3. Reciprocal depression is present in all three inferior leads. Artifact has run lead I off the tracing. Axis is approximately 55°.

CHAPTER 10

Figure 10–9: Nonspecific ST and T wave changes with sagging ST segments less than 1 mm deep and not clearly diagnostic of ischemia. Axis is approximately 42°.
Figure 10–10: Horizontal or slightly downsloping ST depression of up to 2 mm and an abrupt angle with the T wave, all characteristic of myocardial ischemia. There is poor R wave progression in leads V_1 through V_3, raising

161

the question of, but not proving, an old anterior infarction. Axis is approximately 36°.

Figure 10–11: Sagging ST segments in many limb leads but fairly clear straight and horizontal or downsloping depression in leads V_4 through V_6 of greater than 1 mm, compatible with myocardial ischemia. Axis is about 40°.

Figure 10–12: Full 12-lead ECG tracing with, again, widespread ST depression reaching characteristic criteria for myocardial ischemia, most clearly in leads II and V_6. There is J-point elevation in leads V_2 and V_3, but it is not characteristic of acute anterior wall infarction. Axis is approximately 0°.

Index

Note: Page numbers in *italics* refer to illustrations; page numbers followed by t refer to tables.